Vincent (Vince) Perez, world-renowned and award-winning medical illustrator, has dedicated his life to perfecting his work. The hundreds of illustrations that grace this anatomy atlas attest to his passion for the human form and his commitment to its accurate representation. For decades, Vince's work has illuminated the study of anatomy for millions of students and health-care professionals worldwide. In particular, beginning with the first anatomy guide he created for BarCharts in 1994, he has produced guides of the full body as well as of each system in detail, rounding out their extensive *QuickStudy* academic and medical product line with his instructive illustrations. His meticulous rendering of the human body—whether in broad view of the form as a whole or in minute focus of isolated parts and cells—showcases its features with unsurpassed intricacy of detail.

Vince's client list is as impressive as it is diverse, spanning the globe and encompassing the industries of health care, biotechnology, pharmaceuticals, mass media, telecommunications and transportation: ABC TV; British Airways, Ciba-Geigy, Ltd.; Cutter Laboratories; Disney; Lucasfilm, Ltd.; Pacific Bell; Potlatch Corporation; Simon & Schuster; Sterling-Winthrop; Syntex Corporation; Time, Inc.; Wright Medical Technologies; and many more. In addition to the commercial illustrations he produces for his numerous clients, Vince's multimedia art forms have enjoyed—and continue to enjoy—audiences in virtually every corner of the world, from the United States to Europe to Asia. In addition to being featured at the Osaka World's Fair in Japan, his work is showcased in the permanent collections of several world-class institutions, including the Vatican Museum (Vatican City, Italy), the San Francisco Museum of Modern Art and the California Legion of Honor (San Francisco, California), and the National Portrait Gallery (Washington, D.C.).

Always, his art awes and inspires spectators. Awards and accolades galore attest to this fact: Gold Award from the Western Art Director's Club; Award of Excellence from the Rx Club (New York); CA Award of Excellence, Design Annual; Award of Excellence, Mead Show, National Medical Enterprises, Inc.; Fourth Annual LULU Award of Excellence; San Francisco Society of Illustrators Technical Illustration Gold and Silver Awards; and the crowning achievement, two pieces chosen by the Society of Illustrators (New York) for selection among 100 of the best medical illustrations ever produced in the United States.

Born and raised on the East Coast, Vince has lived in California since 1964. Today he divides his time amongst his many beloved pursuits: first and foremost, his art; then his teaching of future artists and his volunteerism in the Alameda, California, community he calls home. A full-tenured professor at the California College of the Arts (CCA), where he has chaired the illustration and drawing programs that he helped develop, Vince instructs students in illustration, life drawing, printmaking, and of course, anatomy. He has also taught anatomy and illustration at the University of California at Berkeley (UCB). He holds a B.F.A. in graphic arts and illustration from Pratt Institute in New York, and an M.F.A. in painting from the California College of Arts & Crafts (now CCA). He also completed graduate work in fine arts at the University of the Americas in Mexico City (Mexico).

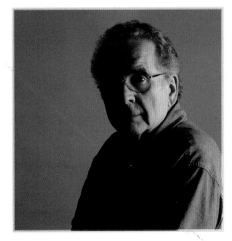

VINCE PEREZ

An artist whose talent truly runs the gamut—he is equally at home creating intricate medical illustrations, cutting-edge graphic designs and whimsical woodcuts—the genius of Vince Perez comes to life on every page of this atlas, and his at-once informative and innovative anatomical renderings are sure to enrich your medical experience at whatever point you are in your education—beginning student awed by the medical universe, seasoned professional seeking further knowledge, or curious layperson expanding a home-health library. No matter, you are sure to find the Perez-illustrated journey to be as instructive as it is unforgettable.

Let Vince's unparalleled representation of the human body illuminate your foray into the world of medicine! (To see a sampling of his work, please visit *www.perezstudio.com*.)

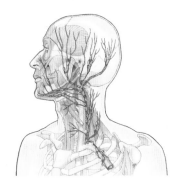

©2006 BarCharts, Inc.
ISBN 13: 9781423201724
ISBN 10: 1423201728

BarCharts and QuickStudy are registered trademarks of BarCharts, Inc.

Publisher: BarCharts, Inc.
6000 Park of Commerce Boulevard, Suite D
Boca Raton, FL 33487
www.quickstudy.com

Artist: Vincent Perez
Images © Vincent Perez / *www.perezstudio.com*
Editing: Lisa Drucker
Proofreading: Kaaren Ashley
Mona Moskowitz
Peter Miller
Art Direction: Rich Marino
Design/Layout: Andre Brisson
Andrea Hutchinson
Dale Nibbe
Latoya Danford

Printed in Thailand

ATLAS *of*
HUMAN ANATOMY

Vincent Perez

BarCharts, Inc.®

Boca Raton, Florida

Contents

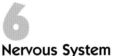

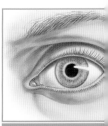

1

SURFACE ANATOMY

FULL BODY

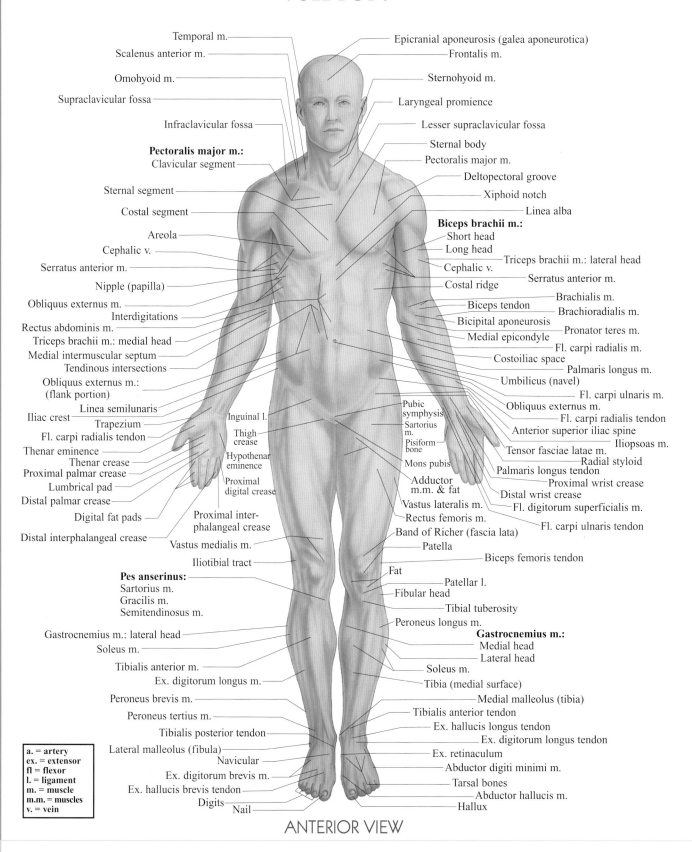

Temporal m.
Scalenus anterior m.
Omohyoid m.
Supraclavicular fossa
Infraclavicular fossa
Pectoralis major m.:
Clavicular segment
Sternal segment
Costal segment
Areola
Cephalic v.
Serratus anterior m.
Nipple (papilla)
Obliquus externus m.
Interdigitations
Rectus abdominis m.
Triceps brachii m.: medial head
Medial intermuscular septum
Tendinous intersections
Obliquus externus m.:
(flank portion)
Linea semilunaris
Iliac crest
Trapezium
Fl. carpi radialis tendon
Thenar eminence
Thenar crease
Proximal palmar crease
Lumbrical pad
Distal palmar crease
Digital fat pads
Distal interphalangeal crease
Vastus medialis m.
Iliotibial tract
Pes anserinus:
Sartorius m.
Gracilis m.
Semitendinosus m.
Gastrocnemius m.: lateral head
Soleus m.
Tibialis anterior m.
Ex. digitorum longus m.
Peroneus brevis m.
Peroneus tertius m.
Tibialis posterior tendon
Lateral malleolus (fibula)
Navicular
Ex. digitorum brevis m.
Ex. hallucis brevis tendon
Digits
Nail

Epicranial aponeurosis (galea aponeurotica)
Frontalis m.
Sternohyoid m.
Laryngeal promience
Lesser supraclavicular fossa
Sternal body
Pectoralis major m.
Deltopectoral groove
Xiphoid notch
Linea alba
Biceps brachii m.:
Short head
Long head
Triceps brachii m.: lateral head
Cephalic v.
Serratus anterior m.
Costal ridge
Brachialis m.
Biceps tendon
Brachioradialis m.
Bicipital aponeurosis
Pronator teres m.
Medial epicondyle
Fl. carpi radialis m.
Costoiliac space
Palmaris longus m.
Umbilicus (navel)
Fl. carpi ulnaris m.
Obliquus externus m.
Fl. carpi radialis tendon
Anterior superior iliac spine
Iliopsoas m.
Tensor fasciae latae m.
Radial styloid
Palmaris longus tendon
Proximal wrist crease
Distal wrist crease
Fl. digitorum superficialis m.
Fl. carpi ulnaris tendon

Inguinal l.
Thigh crease
Hypothenar eminence
Proximal digital crease
Proximal inter-phalangeal crease

Pubic symphysis
Sartorius m.
Pisiform bone
Mons pubis
Adductor m.m. & fat
Vastus lateralis m.
Rectus femoris m.
Band of Richer (fascia lata)
Patella
Biceps femoris tendon
Fat
Patellar l.
Fibular head
Tibial tuberosity
Peroneus longus m.
Gastrocnemius m.:
Medial head
Lateral head
Soleus m.
Tibia (medial surface)
Medial malleolus (tibia)
Tibialis anterior tendon
Ex. hallucis longus tendon
Ex. digitorum longus tendon
Ex. retinaculum
Abductor digiti minimi m.
Tarsal bones
Abductor hallucis m.
Hallux

a. = artery
ex. = extensor
fl = flexor
l. = ligament
m. = muscle
m.m. = muscles
v. = vein

ANTERIOR VIEW

FULL BODY

Epicranial aponeurosis (galea aponeurotica)
Mastoid process
Posterior triangle of neck
Levator scapulae m.
Nuchal ridge
Trapezius m.
Omohyoid m.
Trapezius m.
Acromion (scapula)
7th cervical vertebrae
Spine of scapula
Head of humerus
Rear deltoid m.
Side deltoid m.
Trapezius m.
Infraspinatus m.
Teres minor m.
Teres major m.
Edge of latissimus dorsi m.
[See lateral arm for continuation]
Ribs
Serratus anterior m.
Latissimus dorsi m.
Ribs
Erector spinae m.
Inferior rib margin
Flank fat pad
Gluteus maximus m.
Gluteal fat
Biceps femoris m.: long head
Biceps femoris m.: short head
Semimembranosus m.
Popliteal fossa
Biceps femoris tendon
Head of fibula
Gastrocnemius m.: lateral head
Soleus m.
Peroneus longus m.
Peroneus brevis m.
Tendo calcaneus (Achilles)
Proximal heel crease
Distal heel crease
Fl. hallucis longus m.
Calcaneus
Calcaneal fat pad
Peroneal tendons
Abductor digiti minimi m.

Temporal ridge
Temporal m.
Sternocleidomastoid m.
Masseter m.
Submandibular triangle
Superior neck crease
Thyroid cartilage
Inferior neck crease
Cricoid cartilage & thyroid gland
Clavicular head of sternocleidomastoid m.
Clavicle
Coracoid process (scapula)
Front deltoid m.
Pectoralis major m.
Areola
Nipple
Rectus abdominis m.
Obliquus externus m.: (area of interdigitation)
Costal cartilage
Tendinous intersections
Rectus abdominis m.
Linea semilunaris
Umbilicus
Obliquus externus m.: (flank portion)
Iliac crest
Anterior superior iliac spine
Sartorius m.
Gluteus medius m.
Mons pubis
Tensor fasciae latae m.
Great trochanter (femur)
Rectus femoris m.
Iliotibial tract
Vastus lateralis m.
Quadriceps femoris tendon
Lateral epicondyle of femur
Patella
Iliotibial tract
Fat
Patellar l.
Tibial tuberosity
Ex. digitorum longus m.
Tibialis anterior m.
Peroneus tertius m.
Lateral malleolus (fibula)
Tibialis anterior tendon
Ex. hallucis longus tendon
Ex. hallucis brevis m.
Ex. digitorum brevis m.
5th metatarsal tuberosity
Ex. digitorum longus tendons
Digital fat pads

LATERAL VIEW

3

FULL BODY

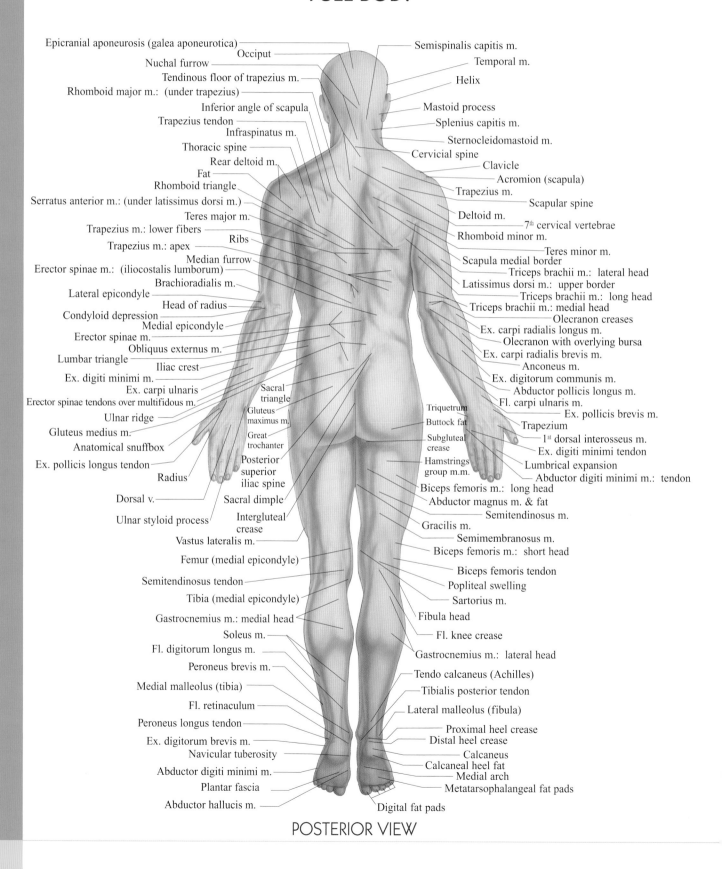

Epicranial aponeurosis (galea aponeurotica)
Occiput
Nuchal furrow
Tendinous floor of trapezius m.
Rhomboid major m.: (under trapezius)
Inferior angle of scapula
Trapezius tendon
Infraspinatus m.
Thoracic spine
Rear deltoid m.
Fat
Rhomboid triangle
Serratus anterior m.: (under latissimus dorsi m.)
Teres major m.
Trapezius m.: lower fibers
Ribs
Trapezius m.: apex
Median furrow
Erector spinae m.: (iliocostalis lumborum)
Brachioradialis m.
Lateral epicondyle
Head of radius
Condyloid depression
Medial epicondyle
Erector spinae m.
Obliquus externus m.
Lumbar triangle
Iliac crest
Ex. digiti minimi m.
Ex. carpi ulnaris
Erector spinae tendons over multifidous m.
Ulnar ridge
Gluteus medius m.
Anatomical snuffbox
Ex. pollicis longus tendon
Radius
Dorsal v.
Ulnar styloid process
Vastus lateralis m.
Femur (medial epicondyle)
Semitendinosus tendon
Tibia (medial epicondyle)
Gastrocnemius m.: medial head
Soleus m.
Fl. digitorum longus m.
Peroneus brevis m.
Medial malleolus (tibia)
Fl. retinaculum
Peroneus longus tendon
Ex. digitorum brevis m.
Navicular tuberosity
Abductor digiti minimi m.
Plantar fascia
Abductor hallucis m.

Sacral triangle
Gluteus maximus m.
Great trochanter
Posterior superior iliac spine
Sacral dimple
Intergluteal crease

Semispinalis capitis m.
Temporal m.
Helix
Mastoid process
Splenius capitis m.
Sternocleidomastoid m.
Cervicial spine
Clavicle
Acromion (scapula)
Trapezius m.
Scapular spine
Deltoid m.
7th cervical vertebrae
Rhomboid minor m.
Teres minor m.
Scapula medial border
Triceps brachii m.: lateral head
Latissimus dorsi m.: upper border
Triceps brachii m.: long head
Triceps brachii m.: medial head
Olecranon creases
Ex. carpi radialis longus m.
Olecranon with overlying bursa
Ex. carpi radialis brevis m.
Anconeus m.
Ex. digitorum communis m.
Abductor pollicis longus m.
Fl. carpi ulnaris m.
Ex. pollicis brevis m.
Trapezium
1st dorsal interosseus m.
Ex. digiti minimi tendon
Lumbrical expansion
Abductor digiti minimi m.: tendon

Triquetrum
Buttock fat
Subgluteal crease
Hamstrings group m.m.
Biceps femoris m.: long head
Abductor magnus m. & fat
Semitendinosus m.
Gracilis m.
Semimembranosus m.
Biceps femoris m.: short head
Biceps femoris tendon
Popliteal swelling
Sartorius m.
Fibula head
Fl. knee crease
Gastrocnemius m.: lateral head
Tendo calcaneus (Achilles)
Tibialis posterior tendon
Lateral malleolus (fibula)
Proximal heel crease
Distal heel crease
Calcaneus
Calcaneal heel fat
Medial arch
Metatarsophalangeal fat pads
Digital fat pads

POSTERIOR VIEW

HEAD

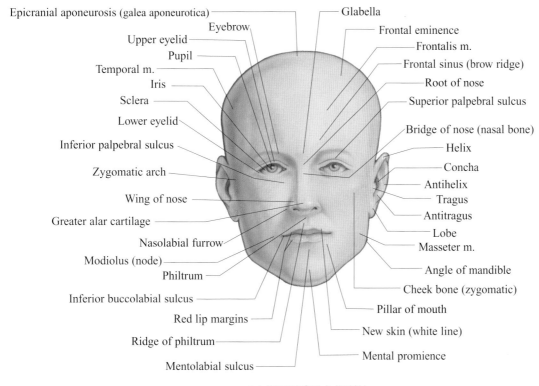

Epicranial aponeurosis (galea aponeurotica)
Eyebrow
Upper eyelid
Pupil
Temporal m.
Iris
Sclera
Lower eyelid
Inferior palpebral sulcus
Zygomatic arch
Wing of nose
Greater alar cartilage
Nasolabial furrow
Modiolus (node)
Philtrum
Inferior buccolabial sulcus
Red lip margins
Ridge of philtrum
Mentolabial sulcus

Glabella
Frontal eminence
Frontalis m.
Frontal sinus (brow ridge)
Root of nose
Superior palpebral sulcus
Bridge of nose (nasal bone)
Helix
Concha
Antihelix
Tragus
Antitragus
Lobe
Masseter m.
Angle of mandible
Cheek bone (zygomatic)
Pillar of mouth
New skin (white line)
Mental promience

ANTERIOR VIEW

EYE

EAR

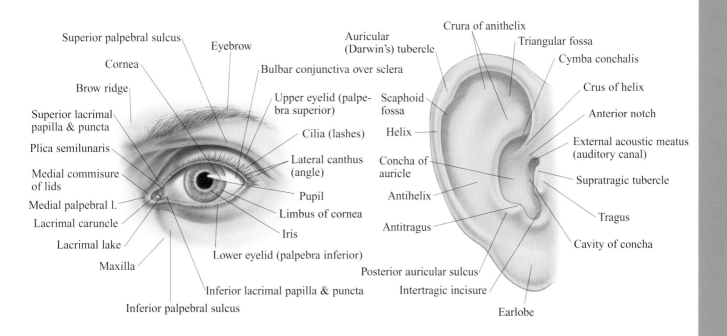

Superior palpebral sulcus
Cornea
Brow ridge
Superior lacrimal
papilla & puncta
Plica semilunaris
Medial commisure
of lids
Medial palpebral l.
Lacrimal caruncle
Lacrimal lake
Maxilla

Eyebrow
Bulbar conjunctiva over sclera
Upper eyelid (palpe-
bra superior)
Cilia (lashes)
Lateral canthus
(angle)
Pupil
Limbus of cornea
Iris
Lower eyelid (palpebra inferior)

Inferior lacrimal papilla & puncta
Inferior palpebral sulcus

Auricular
(Darwin's) tubercle
Bulbar conjunctiva over sclera
Scaphoid
fossa
Helix
Concha of
auricle
Antihelix
Antitragus

Crura of anithelix
Triangular fossa
Cymba conchalis
Crus of helix
Anterior notch
External acoustic meatus
(auditory canal)
Supratragic tubercle
Tragus
Cavity of concha

Posterior auricular sulcus
Intertragic incisure
Earlobe

HEAD

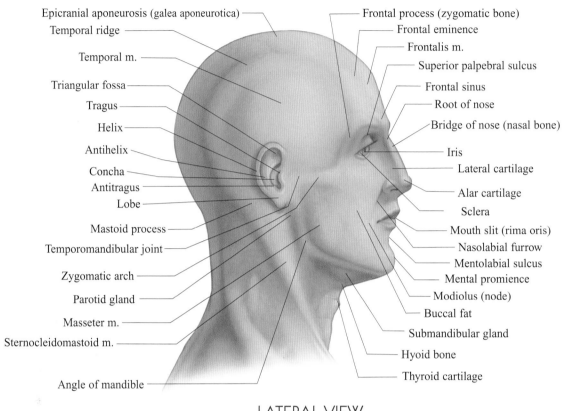

Epicranial aponeurosis (galea aponeurotica)
Temporal ridge
Temporal m.
Triangular fossa
Tragus
Helix
Antihelix
Concha
Antitragus
Lobe
Mastoid process
Temporomandibular joint
Zygomatic arch
Parotid gland
Masseter m.
Sternocleidomastoid m.
Angle of mandible

Frontal process (zygomatic bone)
Frontal eminence
Frontalis m.
Superior palpebral sulcus
Frontal sinus
Root of nose
Bridge of nose (nasal bone)
Iris
Lateral cartilage
Alar cartilage
Sclera
Mouth slit (rima oris)
Nasolabial furrow
Mentolabial sulcus
Mental promince
Modiolus (node)
Buccal fat
Submandibular gland
Hyoid bone
Thyroid cartilage

LATERAL VIEW

MOUTH & NOSE

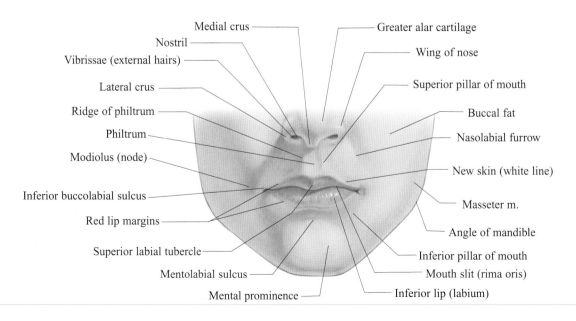

Medial crus
Nostril
Vibrissae (external hairs)
Lateral crus
Ridge of philtrum
Philtrum
Modiolus (node)
Inferior buccolabial sulcus
Red lip margins
Superior labial tubercle
Mentolabial sulcus
Mental prominence

Greater alar cartilage
Wing of nose
Superior pillar of mouth
Buccal fat
Nasolabial furrow
New skin (white line)
Masseter m.
Angle of mandible
Inferior pillar of mouth
Mouth slit (rima oris)
Inferior lip (labium)

RIGHT ARM & HAND

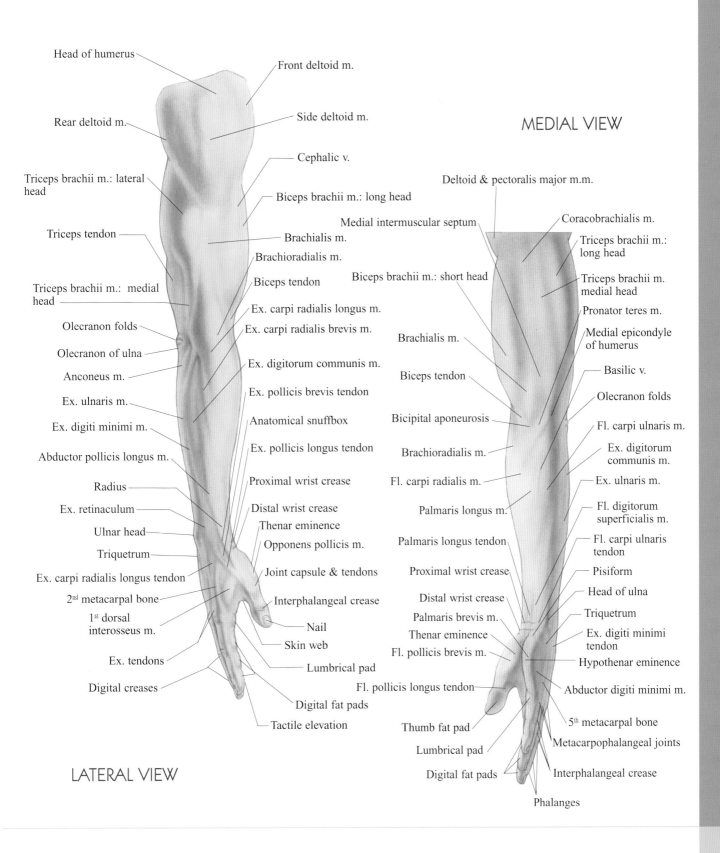

Head of humerus

Rear deltoid m.

Triceps brachii m.: lateral head

Triceps tendon

Triceps brachii m.: medial head

Olecranon folds

Olecranon of ulna

Anconeus m.

Ex. ulnaris m.

Ex. digiti minimi m.

Abductor pollicis longus m.

Radius

Ex. retinaculum

Ulnar head

Triquetrum

Ex. carpi radialis longus tendon

2nd metacarpal bone

1st dorsal interosseus m.

Ex. tendons

Digital creases

Front deltoid m.

Side deltoid m.

Cephalic v.

Biceps brachii m.: long head

Brachialis m.

Brachioradialis m.

Biceps tendon

Ex. carpi radialis longus m.

Ex. carpi radialis brevis m.

Ex. digitorum communis m.

Ex. pollicis brevis tendon

Anatomical snuffbox

Ex. pollicis longus tendon

Proximal wrist crease

Distal wrist crease

Thenar eminence

Opponens pollicis m.

Joint capsule & tendons

Interphalangeal crease

Nail

Skin web

Lumbrical pad

Digital fat pads

Tactile elevation

MEDIAL VIEW

Deltoid & pectoralis major m.m.

Medial intermuscular septum

Biceps brachii m.: short head

Brachialis m.

Biceps tendon

Bicipital aponeurosis

Brachioradialis m.

Fl. carpi radialis m.

Palmaris longus m.

Palmaris longus tendon

Proximal wrist crease

Distal wrist crease

Palmaris brevis m.

Thenar eminence

Fl. pollicis brevis m.

Fl. pollicis longus tendon

Thumb fat pad

Lumbrical pad

Digital fat pads

Coracobrachialis m.

Triceps brachii m.: long head

Triceps brachii m. medial head

Pronator teres m.

Medial epicondyle of humerus

Basilic v.

Olecranon folds

Fl. carpi ulnaris m.

Ex. digitorum communis m.

Ex. ulnaris m.

Fl. digitorum superficialis m.

Fl. carpi ulnaris tendon

Pisiform

Head of ulna

Triquetrum

Ex. digiti minimi tendon

Hypothenar eminence

Abductor digiti minimi m.

5th metacarpal bone

Metacarpophalangeal joints

Interphalangeal crease

Phalanges

LATERAL VIEW

HAND

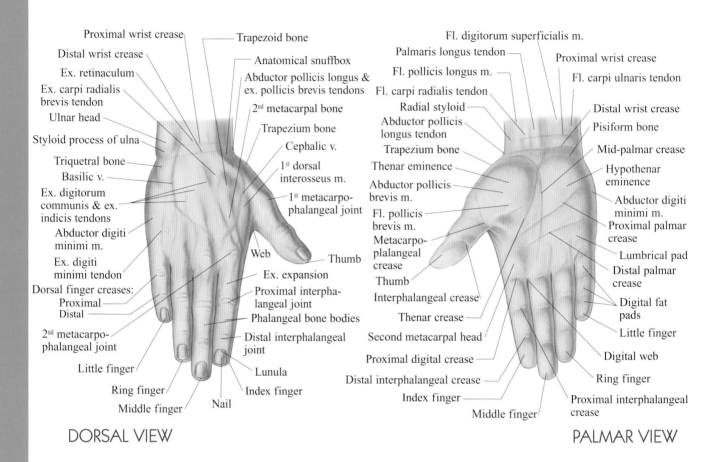

Proximal wrist crease
Distal wrist crease
Ex. retinaculum
Ex. carpi radialis brevis tendon
Ulnar head
Styloid process of ulna
Triquetral bone
Basilic v.
Ex. digitorum communis & ex. indicis tendons
Abductor digiti minimi m.
Ex. digiti minimi tendon
Dorsal finger creases:
Proximal
Distal
2nd metacarpo-phalangeal joint
Little finger
Ring finger
Middle finger

Trapezoid bone
Anatomical snuffbox
Abductor pollicis longus & ex. pollicis brevis tendons
2nd metacarpal bone
Trapezium bone
Cephalic v.
1st dorsal interosseus m.
1st metacarpo-phalangeal joint
Web
Thumb
Ex. expansion
Proximal interpha-langeal joint
Phalangeal bone bodies
Distal interphalangeal joint
Lunula
Nail
Index finger

DORSAL VIEW

Fl. digitorum superficialis m.
Palmaris longus tendon
Fl. pollicis longus m.
Fl. carpi radialis tendon
Radial styloid
Abductor pollicis longus tendon
Trapezium bone
Thenar eminence
Abductor pollicis brevis m.
Fl. pollicis brevis m.
Metacarpo-plalangeal crease
Thumb
Interphalangeal crease
Thenar crease
Second metacarpal head
Proximal digital crease
Distal interphalangeal crease
Index finger
Middle finger

Proximal wrist crease
Fl. carpi ulnaris tendon
Distal wrist crease
Pisiform bone
Mid-palmar crease
Hypothenar eminence
Abductor digiti minimi m.
Proximal palmar crease
Lumbrical pad
Distal palmar crease
Digital fat pads
Little finger
Digital web
Ring finger
Proximal interphalangeal crease

PALMAR VIEW

AXILLA & BREAST

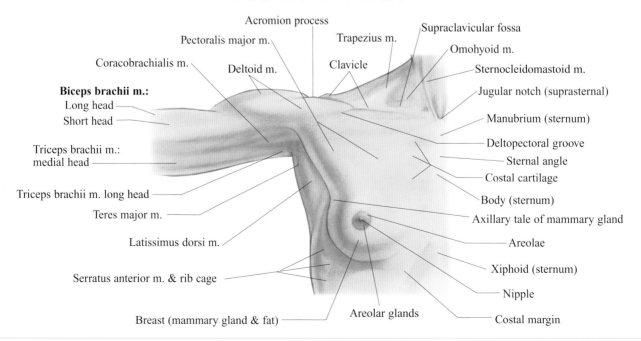

Acromion process
Pectoralis major m.
Coracobrachialis m.
Deltoid m.
Biceps brachii m.:
Long head
Short head
Triceps brachii m.:
medial head
Triceps brachii m. long head
Teres major m.
Latissimus dorsi m.
Serratus anterior m. & rib cage
Breast (mammary gland & fat)

Trapezius m.
Clavicle
Supraclavicular fossa
Omohyoid m.
Sternocleidomastoid m.
Jugular notch (suprasternal)
Manubrium (sternum)
Deltopectoral groove
Sternal angle
Costal cartilage
Body (sternum)
Axillary tale of mammary gland
Areolae
Xiphoid (sternum)
Nipple
Costal margin
Areolar glands

HIPS

FEMALE VIEW

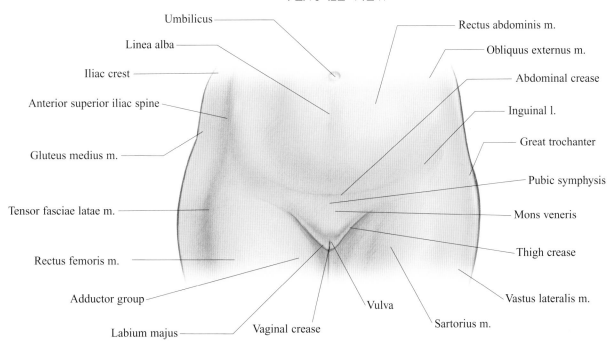

Umbilicus

Linea alba

Iliac crest

Anterior superior iliac spine

Gluteus medius m.

Tensor fasciae latae m.

Rectus femoris m.

Adductor group

Labium majus

Vaginal crease

Vulva

Sartorius m.

Rectus abdominis m.

Obliquus externus m.

Abdominal crease

Inguinal l.

Great trochanter

Pubic symphysis

Mons veneris

Thigh crease

Vastus lateralis m.

MALE VIEW

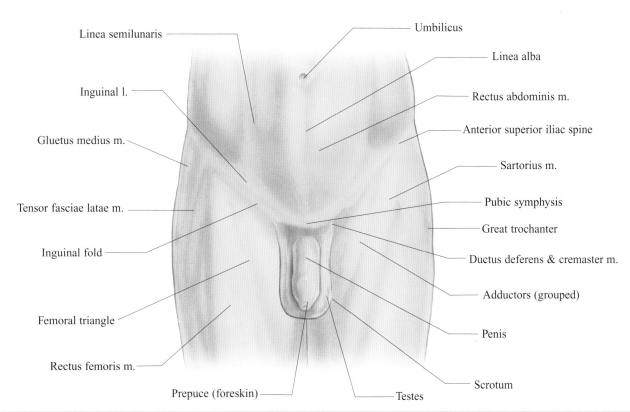

Linea semilunaris

Inguinal l.

Gluetus medius m.

Tensor fasciae latae m.

Inguinal fold

Femoral triangle

Rectus femoris m.

Prepuce (foreskin)

Testes

Umbilicus

Linea alba

Rectus abdominis m.

Anterior superior iliac spine

Sartorius m.

Pubic symphysis

Great trochanter

Ductus deferens & cremaster m.

Adductors (grouped)

Penis

Scrotum

LEG & FOOT

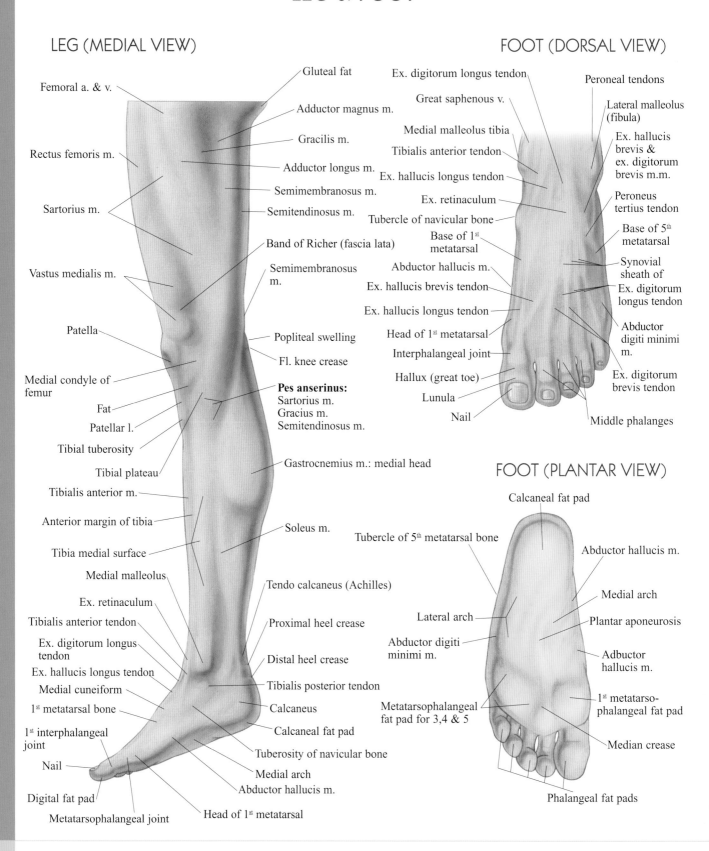

LEG (MEDIAL VIEW)

Femoral a. & v.

Rectus femoris m.

Sartorius m.

Vastus medialis m.

Patella

Medial condyle of femur

Fat

Patellar l.

Tibial tuberosity

Tibial plateau

Tibialis anterior m.

Anterior margin of tibia

Tibia medial surface

Medial malleolus

Ex. retinaculum

Tibialis anterior tendon

Ex. digitorum longus tendon

Ex. hallucis longus tendon

Medial cuneiform

1st metatarsal bone

1st interphalangeal joint

Nail

Digital fat pad

Metatarsophalangeal joint

Gluteal fat

Adductor magnus m.

Gracilis m.

Adductor longus m.

Semimembranosus m.

Semitendinosus m.

Band of Richer (fascia lata)

Semimembranosus m.

Popliteal swelling

Fl. knee crease

Pes anserinus:
Sartorius m.
Gracius m.
Semitendinosus m.

Gastrocnemius m.: medial head

Soleus m.

Tendo calcaneus (Achilles)

Proximal heel crease

Distal heel crease

Tibialis posterior tendon

Calcaneus

Calcaneal fat pad

Tuberosity of navicular bone

Medial arch

Abductor hallucis m.

Head of 1st metatarsal

FOOT (DORSAL VIEW)

Ex. digitorum longus tendon

Great saphenous v.

Medial malleolus tibia

Tibialis anterior tendon

Ex. hallucis longus tendon

Ex. retinaculum

Tubercle of navicular bone

Base of 1st metatarsal

Abductor hallucis m.

Ex. hallucis brevis tendon

Ex. hallucis longus tendon

Head of 1st metatarsal

Interphalangeal joint

Hallux (great toe)

Lunula

Nail

Peroneal tendons

Lateral malleolus (fibula)

Ex. hallucis brevis & ex. digitorum brevis m.m.

Peroneus tertius tendon

Base of 5th metatarsal

Synovial sheath of Ex. digitorum longus tendon

Abductor digiti minimi m.

Ex. digitorum brevis tendon

Middle phalanges

FOOT (PLANTAR VIEW)

Calcaneal fat pad

Tubercle of 5th metatarsal bone

Lateral arch

Abductor digiti minimi m.

Metatarsophalangeal fat pad for 3,4 & 5

Abductor hallucis m.

Medial arch

Plantar aponeurosis

Adbuctor hallucis m.

1st metatarso-phalangeal fat pad

Median crease

Phalangeal fat pads

NOTES

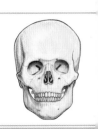

2

SKELETAL SYSTEM

FEMALE SKELETON
ANTERIOR VIEW

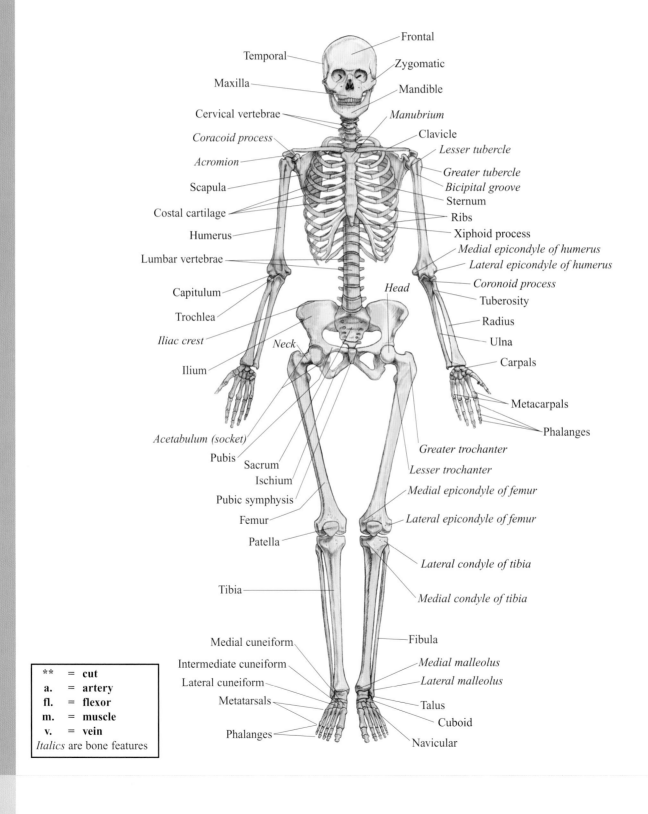

Frontal
Temporal
Zygomatic
Maxilla
Mandible
Cervical vertebrae
Manubrium
Clavicle
Coracoid process
Lesser tubercle
Acromion
Greater tubercle
Scapula
Bicipital groove
Sternum
Costal cartilage
Ribs
Humerus
Xiphoid process
Medial epicondyle of humerus
Lumbar vertebrae
Lateral epicondyle of humerus
Coronoid process
Capitulum
Head
Tuberosity
Trochlea
Radius
Iliac crest
Neck
Ulna
Ilium
Carpals
Metacarpals
Phalanges
Acetabulum (socket)
Pubis
Greater trochanter
Sacrum
Lesser trochanter
Ischium
Medial epicondyle of femur
Pubic symphysis
Femur
Lateral epicondyle of femur
Patella
Lateral condyle of tibia
Medial condyle of tibia
Tibia
Fibula
Medial cuneiform
Medial malleolus
Intermediate cuneiform
Lateral malleolus
Lateral cuneiform
Metatarsals
Talus
Cuboid
Phalanges
Navicular

**	=	**cut**
a.	=	**artery**
fl.	=	**flexor**
m.	=	**muscle**
v.	=	**vein**

Italics are bone features

MALE SKELETON
ANTERIOR VIEW

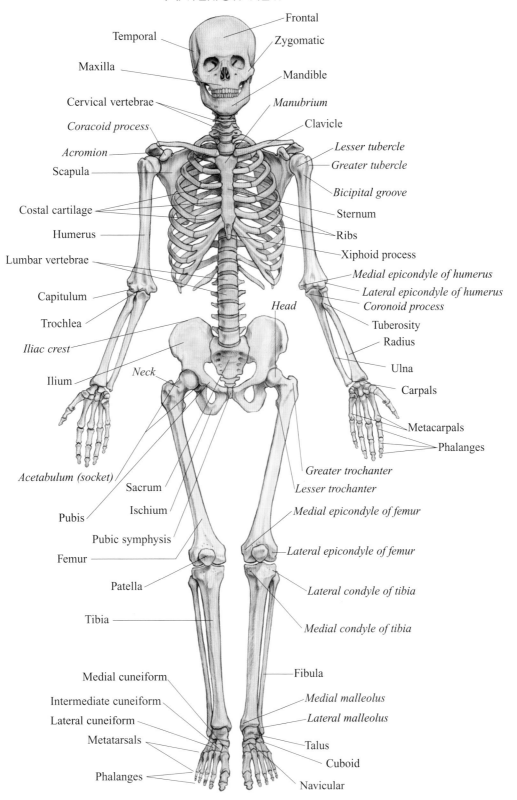

Temporal

Maxilla

Cervical vertebrae

Coracoid process

Acromion

Scapula

Costal cartilage

Humerus

Lumbar vertebrae

Capitulum

Trochlea

Iliac crest

Ilium

Acetabulum (socket)

Pubis

Neck

Sacrum

Ischium

Pubic symphysis

Femur

Patella

Tibia

Medial cuneiform

Intermediate cuneiform

Lateral cuneiform

Metatarsals

Phalanges

Frontal

Zygomatic

Mandible

Manubrium

Clavicle

Lesser tubercle

Greater tubercle

Bicipital groove

Sternum

Ribs

Xiphoid process

Medial epicondyle of humerus

Lateral epicondyle of humerus

Coronoid process

Head

Tuberosity

Radius

Ulna

Carpals

Metacarpals

Phalanges

Greater trochanter

Lesser trochanter

Medial epicondyle of femur

Lateral epicondyle of femur

Lateral condyle of tibia

Medial condyle of tibia

Fibula

Medial malleolus

Lateral malleolus

Talus

Cuboid

Navicular

SKELETON
LATERAL VIEW

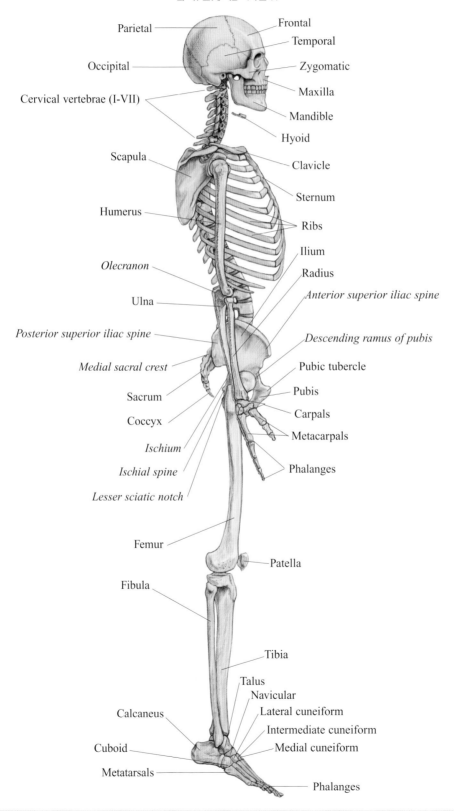

Parietal

Occipital

Cervical vertebrae (I-VII)

Scapula

Humerus

Olecranon

Ulna

Posterior superior iliac spine

Medial sacral crest

Sacrum

Coccyx

Ischium

Ischial spine

Lesser sciatic notch

Femur

Fibula

Calcaneus

Cuboid

Metatarsals

Frontal

Temporal

Zygomatic

Maxilla

Mandible

Hyoid

Clavicle

Sternum

Ribs

Ilium

Radius

Anterior superior iliac spine

Descending ramus of pubis

Pubic tubercle

Pubis

Carpals

Metacarpals

Phalanges

Patella

Tibia

Talus

Navicular

Lateral cuneiform

Intermediate cuneiform

Medial cuneiform

Phalanges

SKELETON
POSTERIOR VIEW

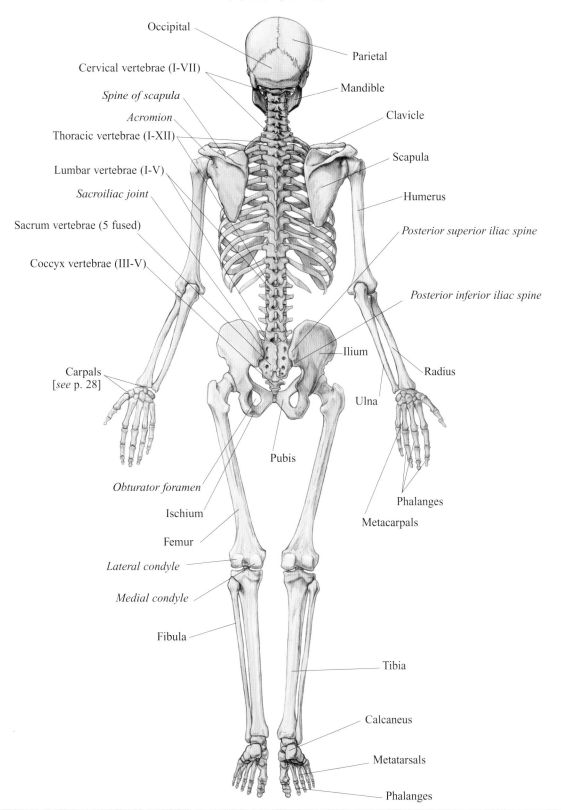

Occipital

Cervical vertebrae (I-VII)

Spine of scapula

Acromion

Thoracic vertebrae (I-XII)

Lumbar vertebrae (I-V)

Sacroiliac joint

Sacrum vertebrae (5 fused)

Coccyx vertebrae (III-V)

Carpals
[*see* p. 28]

Obturator foramen

Ischium

Femur

Lateral condyle

Medial condyle

Fibula

Parietal

Mandible

Clavicle

Scapula

Humerus

Posterior superior iliac spine

Posterior inferior iliac spine

Ilium

Radius

Ulna

Phalanges

Metacarpals

Pubis

Tibia

Calcaneus

Metatarsals

Phalanges

VERTEBRAL COLUMN
LATERAL VIEW

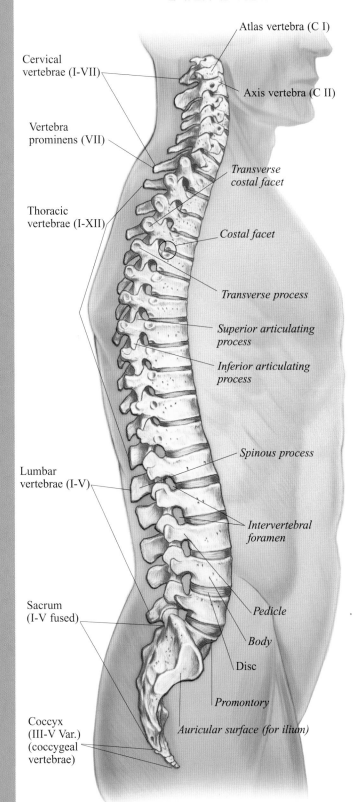

Atlas vertebra (C I)

Cervical vertebrae (I-VII)

Axis vertebra (C II)

Vertebra prominens (VII)

Transverse costal facet

Thoracic vertebrae (I-XII)

Costal facet

Transverse process

Superior articulating process

Inferior articulating process

Spinous process

Lumbar vertebrae (I-V)

Intervertebral foramen

Sacrum (I-V fused)

Pedicle

Body

Disc

Coccyx (III-V Var.) (coccygeal vertebrae)

Promontory

Auricular surface (for ilium)

LUMBAR VERTEBRA
SUPERIOR VIEW

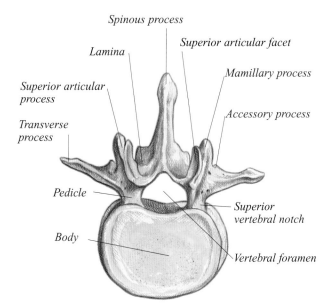

Spinous process

Lamina

Superior articular facet

Mamillary process

Superior articular process

Accessory process

Transverse process

Pedicle

Body

Superior vertebral notch

Vertebral foramen

CERVICAL VERTEBRAE
POSTERIOR VIEW

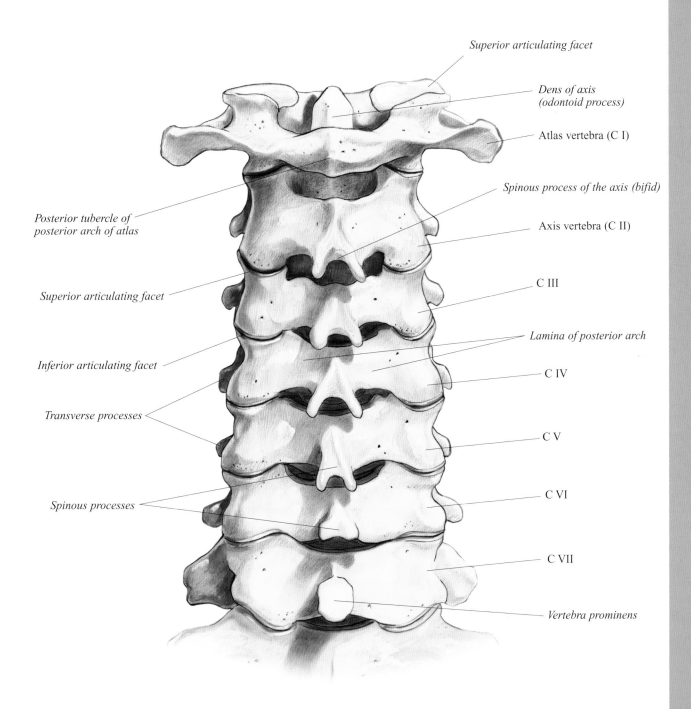

Superior articulating facet

Dens of axis
(odontoid process)

Atlas vertebra (C I)

Spinous process of the axis (bifid)

Axis vertebra (C II)

C III

Lamina of posterior arch

C IV

C V

C VI

C VII

Vertebra prominens

Posterior tubercle of
posterior arch of atlas

Superior articulating facet

Inferior articulating facet

Transverse processes

Spinous processes

LUMBAR VERTEBRAE
POSTERIOR VIEW

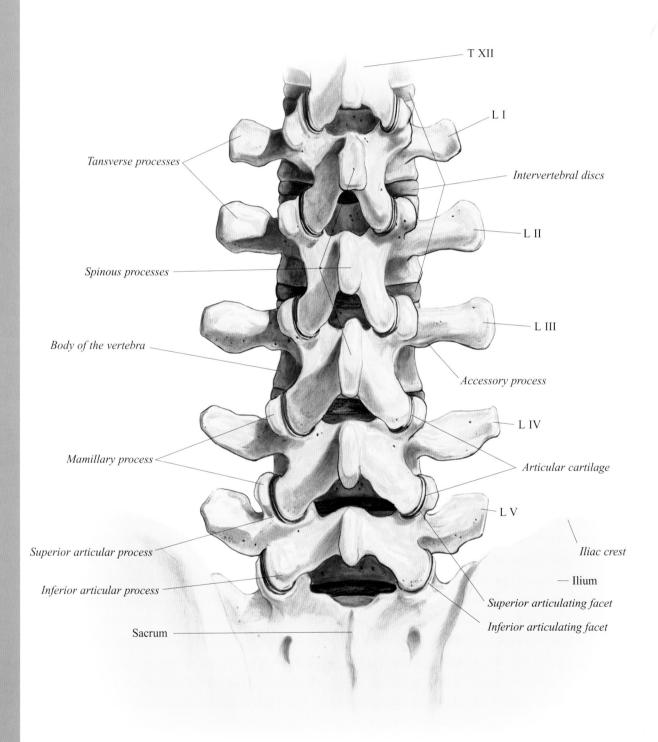

T XII

L I

Intervertebral discs

Tansverse processes

L II

Spinous processes

L III

Body of the vertebra

Accessory process

L IV

Mamillary process

Articular cartilage

L V

Superior articular process

Iliac crest

Ilium

Inferior articular process

Superior articulating facet

Inferior articulating facet

Sacrum

SKULL

LATERAL VIEW

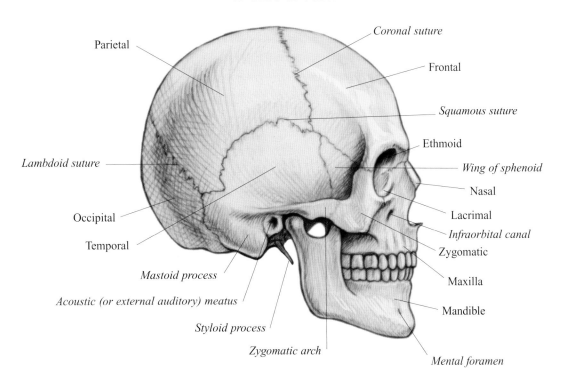

Parietal

Coronal suture

Frontal

Squamous suture

Ethmoid

Wing of sphenoid

Lambdoid suture

Nasal

Lacrimal

Infraorbital canal

Zygomatic

Occipital

Temporal

Maxilla

Mastoid process

Mandible

Acoustic (or external auditory) meatus

Styloid process

Mental foramen

Zygomatic arch

MEDIAN (SAGITTAL) SECTION

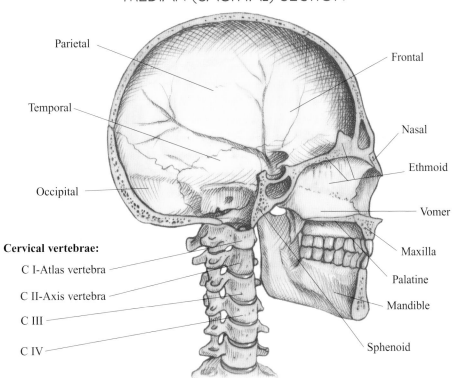

Parietal

Frontal

Temporal

Nasal

Ethmoid

Occipital

Vomer

Cervical vertebrae:

C I-Atlas vertebra

Maxilla

C II-Axis vertebra

Palatine

C III

Mandible

C IV

Sphenoid

SKULL
ANTERIOR VIEW

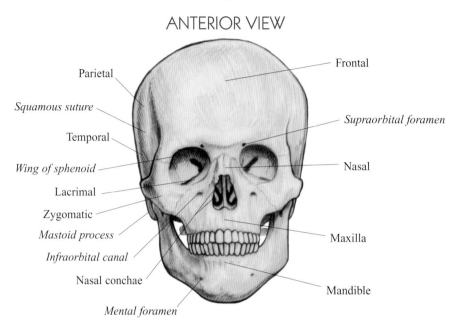

Parietal

Squamous suture

Temporal

Wing of sphenoid

Lacrimal

Zygomatic

Mastoid process

Infraorbital canal

Nasal conchae

Mental foramen

Frontal

Supraorbital foramen

Nasal

Maxilla

Mandible

SKULL
INFERIOR VIEW

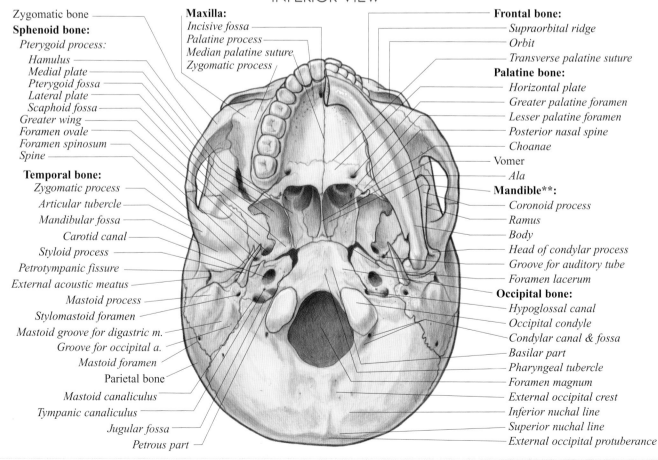

Zygomatic bone

Sphenoid bone:
  Pterygoid process:
    Hamulus
    Medial plate
    Pterygoid fossa
    Lateral plate
    Scaphoid fossa
  Greater wing
  Foramen ovale
  Foramen spinosum
  Spine

Temporal bone:
  Zygomatic process
  Articular tubercle
  Mandibular fossa
  Carotid canal
  Styloid process
  Petrotympanic fissure
  External acoustic meatus
  Mastoid process
  Stylomastoid foramen
  Mastoid groove for digastric m.
  Groove for occipital a.
  Mastoid foramen
  Parietal bone
  Mastoid canaliculus
  Tympanic canaliculus
  Jugular fossa
  Petrous part

Maxilla:
Incisive fossa
Palatine process
Median palatine suture
Zygomatic process

Frontal bone:
  Supraorbital ridge
  Orbit
  Transverse palatine suture
Palatine bone:
  Horizontal plate
  Greater palatine foramen
  Lesser palatine foramen
  Posterior nasal spine
  Choanae
  Vomer
  Ala
Mandible**:
  Coronoid process
  Ramus
  Body
  Head of condylar process
  Groove for auditory tube
  Foramen lacerum
Occipital bone:
  Hypoglossal canal
  Occipital condyle
  Condylar canal & fossa
  Basilar part
  Pharyngeal tubercle
  Foramen magnum
  External occipital crest
  Inferior nuchal line
  Superior nuchal line
  External occipital protuberance

ANTERIOR SKULL & CUT CERVICAL VERTEBRAE
POSTERIOR VIEW CORONAL SECTION

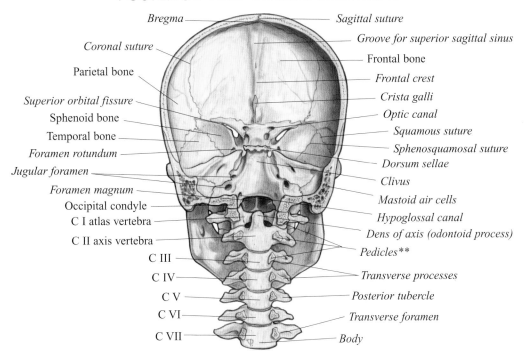

Bregma — Sagittal suture
Coronal suture — Groove for superior sagittal sinus
Parietal bone — Frontal bone
— Frontal crest
Superior orbital fissure — Crista galli
Sphenoid bone — Optic canal
Temporal bone — Squamous suture
Foramen rotundum — Sphenosquamosal suture
Jugular foramen — Dorsum sellae
— Clivus
Foramen magnum — Mastoid air cells
Occipital condyle — Hypoglossal canal
C I atlas vertebra — Dens of axis (odontoid process)
C II axis vertebra — Pedicles**
C III —
C IV — Transverse processes
C V — Posterior tubercle
C VI — Transverse foramen
C VII — Body

SKULL
POSTERIOR VIEW CORONAL SECTION

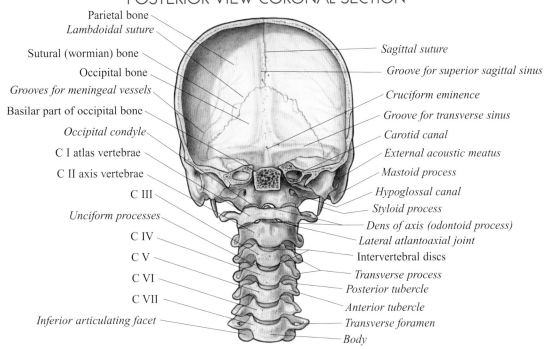

Parietal bone —
Lambdoidal suture —
Sutural (wormian) bone — Sagittal suture
Occipital bone — Groove for superior sagittal sinus
Grooves for meningeal vessels — Cruciform eminence
Basilar part of occipital bone — Groove for transverse sinus
Occipital condyle — Carotid canal
C I atlas vertebrae — External acoustic meatus
C II axis vertebrae — Mastoid process
C III — Hypoglossal canal
Unciform processes — Styloid process
C IV — Dens of axis (odontoid process)
C V — Lateral atlantoaxial joint
— Intervertebral discs
C VI — Transverse process
C VII — Posterior tubercle
— Anterior tubercle
Inferior articulating facet — Transverse foramen
— Body

CERVICAL VERTEBRAE
ANTERIOR VIEW

CLAVICLE
SUPERIOR VIEW

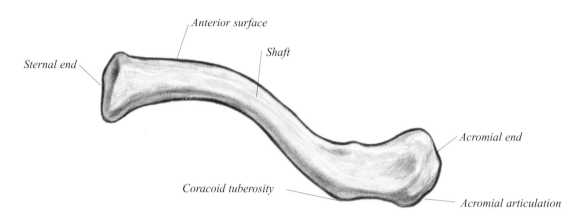

Anterior surface

Shaft

Sternal end

Acromial end

Coracoid tuberosity

Acromial articulation

CLAVICLE
INFERIOR VIEW

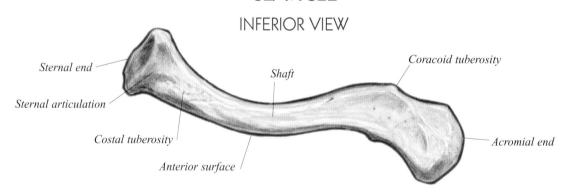

Sternal end

Coracoid tuberosity

Sternal articulation

Shaft

Costal tuberosity

Acromial end

Anterior surface

HYOID BONE

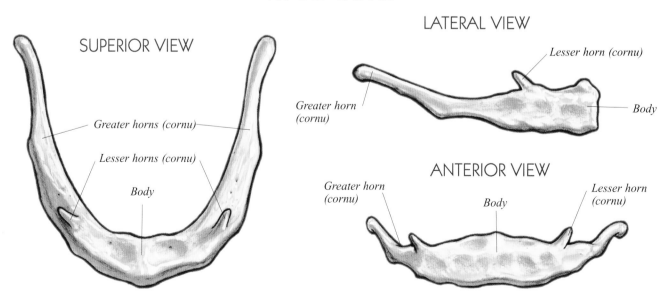

LATERAL VIEW

Lesser horn (cornu)

Greater horn
(cornu)

Body

SUPERIOR VIEW

Greater horns (cornu)

Lesser horns (cornu)

Body

ANTERIOR VIEW

Greater horn
(cornu)

Body

Lesser horn
(cornu)

SCAPULA
ANTERIOR VIEW

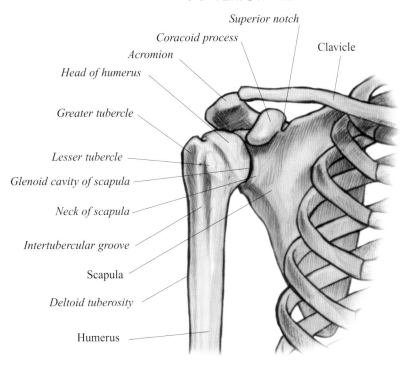

Superior notch

Coracoid process

Acromion

Clavicle

Head of humerus

Greater tubercle

Lesser tubercle

Glenoid cavity of scapula

Neck of scapula

Intertubercular groove

Scapula

Deltoid tuberosity

Humerus

SCAPULA
POSTERIOR VIEW

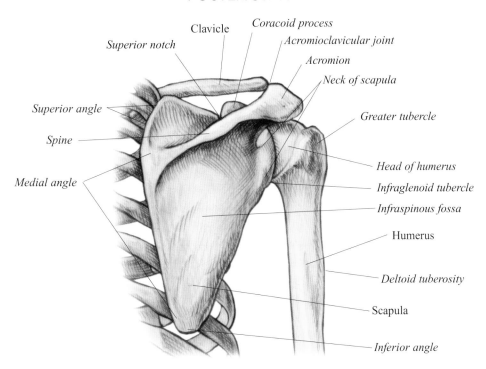

Clavicle

Coracoid process

Superior notch

Acromioclavicular joint

Acromion

Neck of scapula

Superior angle

Greater tubercle

Spine

Head of humerus

Medial angle

Infraglenoid tubercle

Infraspinous fossa

Humerus

Deltoid tuberosity

Scapula

Inferior angle

THORACIC BONES

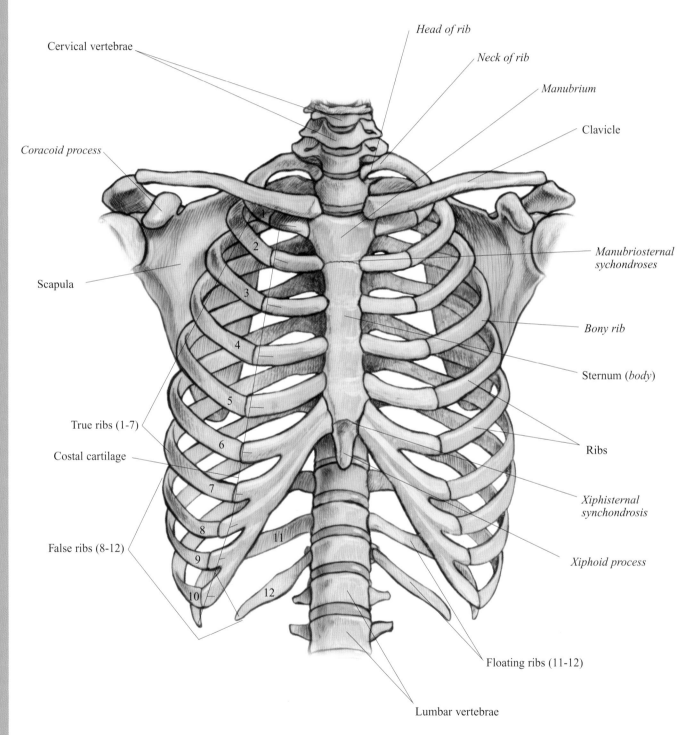

Cervical vertebrae

Head of rib

Neck of rib

Manubrium

Clavicle

Coracoid process

Scapula

Manubriosternal sychondroses

Bony rib

Sternum (*body*)

True ribs (1-7)

Costal cartilage

Ribs

Xiphisternal synchondrosis

False ribs (8-12)

Xiphoid process

Floating ribs (11-12)

Lumbar vertebrae

1
2
3
4
5
6
7
8
9
10
11
12

ANTERIOR VIEW

LEFT HIP BONE
ANTERIOR VIEW

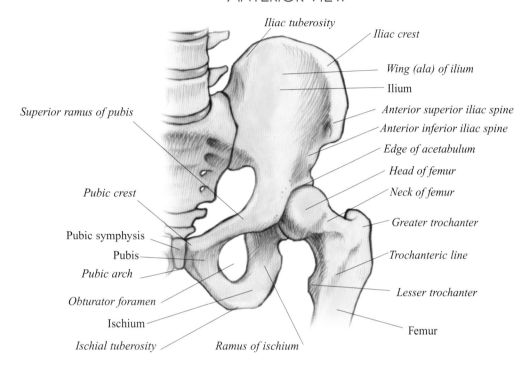

Iliac tuberosity

Iliac crest

Wing (ala) of ilium

Ilium

Anterior superior iliac spine

Anterior inferior iliac spine

Edge of acetabulum

Head of femur

Neck of femur

Greater trochanter

Trochanteric line

Lesser trochanter

Femur

Superior ramus of pubis

Pubic crest

Pubic symphysis

Pubis

Pubic arch

Obturator foramen

Ischium

Ischial tuberosity

Ramus of ischium

LEFT HIP BONE
POSTERIOR VIEW

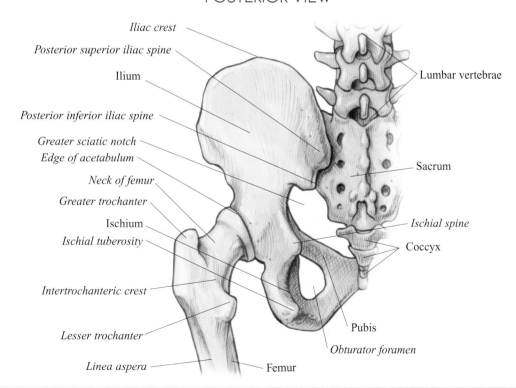

Iliac crest

Posterior superior iliac spine

Ilium

Posterior inferior iliac spine

Greater sciatic notch

Edge of acetabulum

Neck of femur

Greater trochanter

Ischium

Ischial tuberosity

Intertrochanteric crest

Lesser trochanter

Linea aspera

Femur

Lumbar vertebrae

Sacrum

Ischial spine

Coccyx

Pubis

Obturator foramen

SKELETAL SYSTEM

ELBOWS

ANTERIOR VIEW

POSTERIOR VIEW

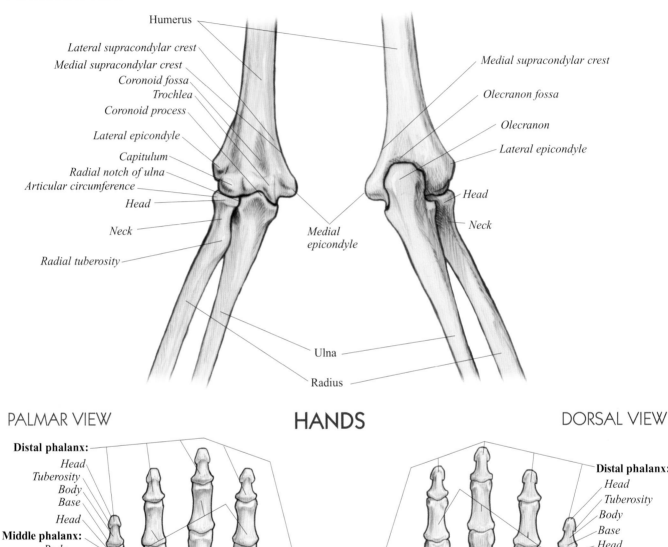

Humerus

Lateral supracondylar crest
Medial supracondylar crest
Coronoid fossa
Trochlea
Coronoid process

Lateral epicondyle

Capitulum
Radial notch of ulna
Articular circumference
Head

Neck

Radial tuberosity

Medial epicondyle

Medial supracondylar crest

Olecranon fossa

Olecranon

Lateral epicondyle

Head

Neck

Ulna

Radius

HANDS

PALMAR VIEW

DORSAL VIEW

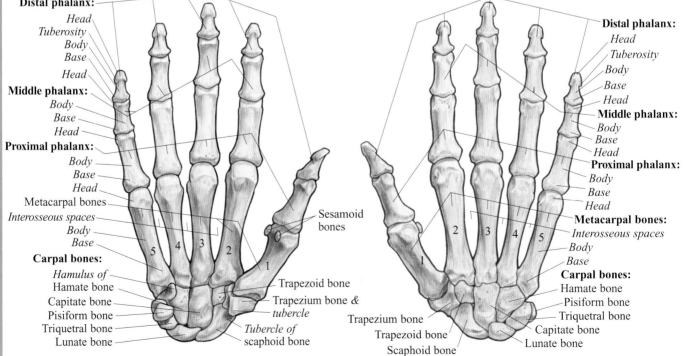

Distal phalanx:
Head
Tuberosity
Body
Base
Head
Middle phalanx:
Body
Base
Head
Proximal phalanx:
Body
Base
Head
Metacarpal bones
Interosseous spaces
Body
Base
Carpal bones:
Hamulus of
Hamate bone
Capitate bone
Pisiform bone
Triquetral bone
Lunate bone

5 4 3 2 0

1

Sesamoid bones

Trapezoid bone

Trapezium bone & tubercle

Tubercle of scaphoid bone

Distal phalanx:
Head
Tuberosity
Body
Base
Head
Middle phalanx:
Body
Base
Head
Proximal phalanx:
Body
Base
Head
Metacarpal bones:
Interosseous spaces
Body
Base
Carpal bones:
Hamate bone
Pisiform bone
Triquetral bone
Capitate bone
Lunate bone

2 3 4 5

1

Trapezium bone
Trapezoid bone
Scaphoid bone

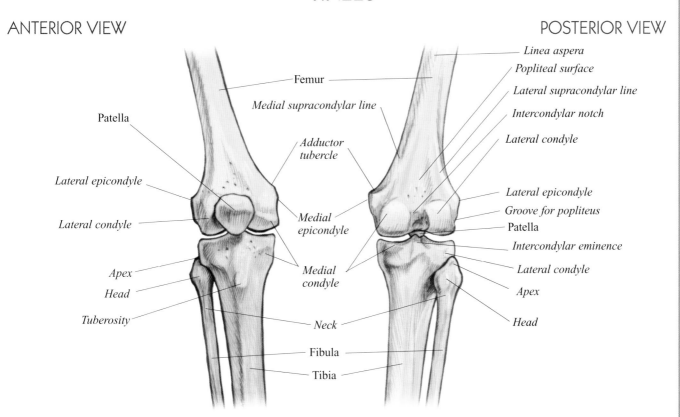

KNEES

ANTERIOR VIEW

POSTERIOR VIEW

Femur

Medial supracondylar line

Patella

Adductor
tubercle

Lateral epicondyle

Lateral condyle

Medial
epicondyle

Apex

Head

Medial
condyle

Tuberosity

Neck

Fibula

Tibia

Linea aspera

Popliteal surface

Lateral supracondylar line

Intercondylar notch

Lateral condyle

Lateral epicondyle

Groove for popliteus

Patella

Intercondylar eminence

Lateral condyle

Apex

Head

PLANTAR VIEW

FEET

DORSAL VIEW

Tuberosity
Base
Head
Body
Base
Sesamoid bones:
Lateral
Medial
Head
Body
Base
**Cuneiform
bones:**
Medial
Intermediate
Lateral
Navicular bone
Tuberosity
Transverse
tarsal joint
Talus:
Head
Posterior process
Medial tubercle
Lateral tubercle

Phalanges:
Distal
Middle
Proximal

Metatarsal bones

Tarsometatarsal joint

Tuberosity of 5th metatarsal

Cuboid bone:

Groove for peroneus longus

Tuberosity

Calcaneus:

Sustenaculum tali
Peroneal trochlea
Groove for fl. hallucis
longus tendon
Lateral process
Medial process
Tuberosity

Phalanges:
Distal
Middle
Proximal

Metatarsal bones

Tarsometatarsal joint

Cuneiform bones:
Medial
Intermediate
Lateral
Navicular bone
Tuberosity
Head
Neck
Trochlea
Groove for fl. hallucis
longus tendon
Talus:
Medial tubercle
Lateral tubercle

Tuberosity
Base
Head
Base
Head
Body
Base
Head
Body
Base
Tuberosity
Cuboid bone
Transverse
tarsal joint
Calcaneus:
Peroneal trochlea
Body

BONE STRUCTURE

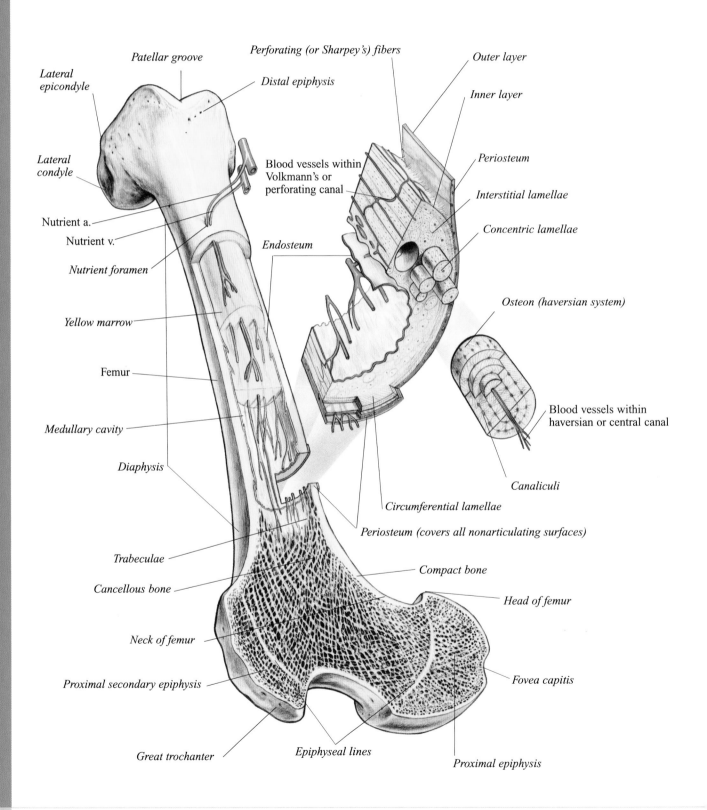

Patellar groove

Lateral epicondyle

Perforating (or Sharpey's) fibers

Distal epiphysis

Outer layer

Inner layer

Periosteum

Interstitial lamellae

Lateral condyle

Blood vessels within Volkmann's or perforating canal

Concentric lamellae

Nutrient a.

Nutrient v.

Nutrient foramen

Endosteum

Osteon (haversian system)

Yellow marrow

Femur

Blood vessels within haversian or central canal

Medullary cavity

Diaphysis

Canaliculi

Circumferential lamellae

Periosteum (covers all nonarticulating surfaces)

Trabeculae

Compact bone

Cancellous bone

Head of femur

Neck of femur

Proximal secondary epiphysis

Fovea capitis

Great trochanter

Epiphyseal lines

Proximal epiphysis

NOTES

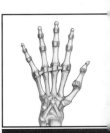

3

JOINTS & LIGAMENTS

JOINTS & LIGAMENTS

SPINE

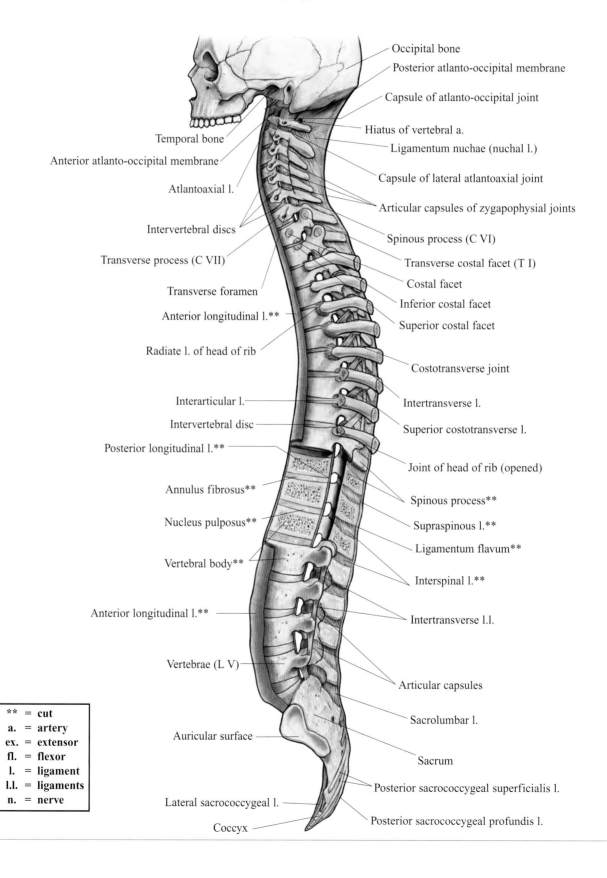

Occipital bone

Posterior atlanto-occipital membrane

Capsule of atlanto-occipital joint

Hiatus of vertebral a.

Ligamentum nuchae (nuchal l.)

Capsule of lateral atlantoaxial joint

Articular capsules of zygapophysial joints

Spinous process (C VI)

Transverse costal facet (T I)

Costal facet

Inferior costal facet

Superior costal facet

Costotransverse joint

Intertransverse l.

Superior costotransverse l.

Joint of head of rib (opened)

Spinous process**

Supraspinous l.**

Ligamentum flavum**

Interspinal l.**

Intertransverse l.l.

Articular capsules

Sacrolumbar l.

Sacrum

Posterior sacrococcygeal superficialis l.

Posterior sacrococcygeal profundis l.

Temporal bone

Anterior atlanto-occipital membrane

Atlantoaxial l.

Intervertebral discs

Transverse process (C VII)

Transverse foramen

Anterior longitudinal l.**

Radiate l. of head of rib

Interarticular l.

Intervertebral disc

Posterior longitudinal l.**

Annulus fibrosus**

Nucleus pulposus**

Vertebral body**

Anterior longitudinal l.**

Vertebrae (L V)

Auricular surface

Lateral sacrococcygeal l.

Coccyx

**	=	cut
a.	=	artery
ex.	=	extensor
fl.	=	flexor
l.	=	ligament
l.l.	=	ligaments
n.	=	nerve

TEMPOROMANDIBULAR & HYOID

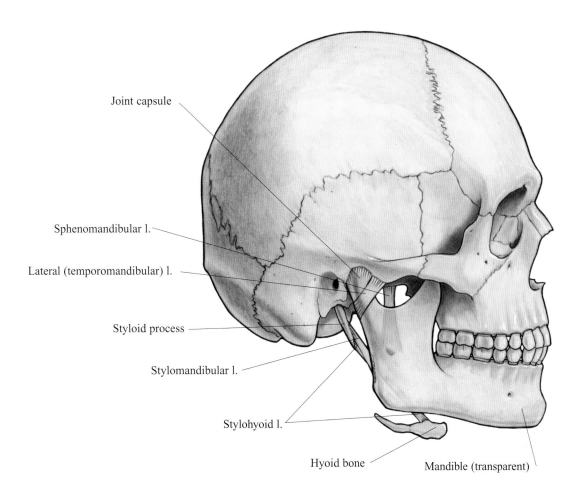

Joint capsule

Sphenomandibular l.

Lateral (temporomandibular) l.

Styloid process

Stylomandibular l.

Stylohyoid l.

Hyoid bone

Mandible (transparent)

TEMPOROMANDIBULAR JOINT

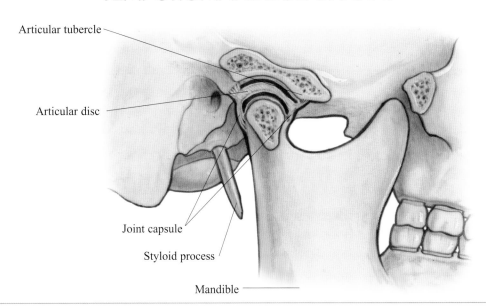

Articular tubercle

Articular disc

Joint capsule

Styloid process

Mandible

JOINTS & LIGAMENTS

CRANIOCERVICAL

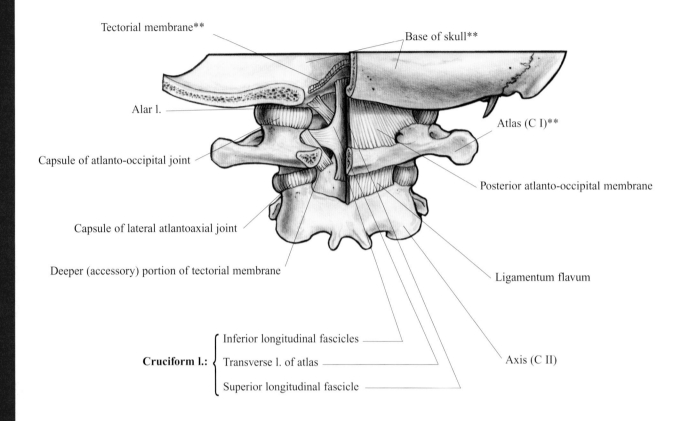

Tectorial membrane**

Base of skull**

Alar l.

Atlas (C I)**

Capsule of atlanto-occipital joint

Posterior atlanto-occipital membrane

Capsule of lateral atlantoaxial joint

Deeper (accessory) portion of tectorial membrane

Ligamentum flavum

Cruciform l.:
- Inferior longitudinal fascicles
- Transverse l. of atlas
- Superior longitudinal fascicle

Axis (C II)

STERNOCLAVICULAR & SHOULDER

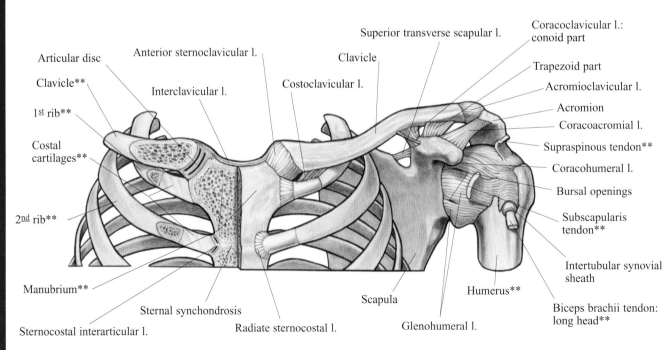

Articular disc

Anterior sternoclavicular l.

Superior transverse scapular l.

Coracoclavicular l.: conoid part

Clavicle**

Clavicle

Trapezoid part

1st rib**

Interclavicular l.

Costoclavicular l.

Acromioclavicular l.

Costal cartilages**

Acromion

Coracoacromial l.

Supraspinous tendon**

Coracohumeral l.

2nd rib**

Bursal openings

Subscapularis tendon**

Intertubular synovial sheath

Manubrium**

Sternal synchondrosis

Radiate sternocostal l.

Scapula

Glenohumeral l.

Humerus**

Biceps brachii tendon: long head**

Sternocostal interarticular l.

ELBOW

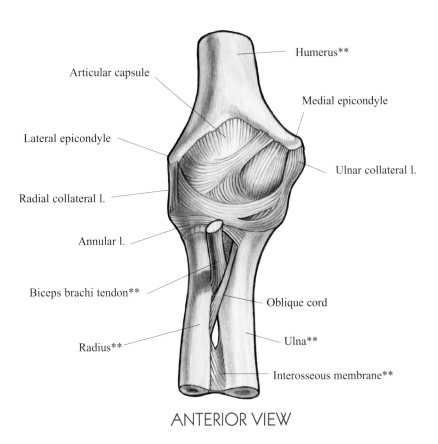

Humerus**

Articular capsule

Medial epicondyle

Lateral epicondyle

Ulnar collateral l.

Radial collateral l.

Annular l.

Biceps brachi tendon**

Oblique cord

Radius**

Ulna**

Interosseous membrane**

ANTERIOR VIEW

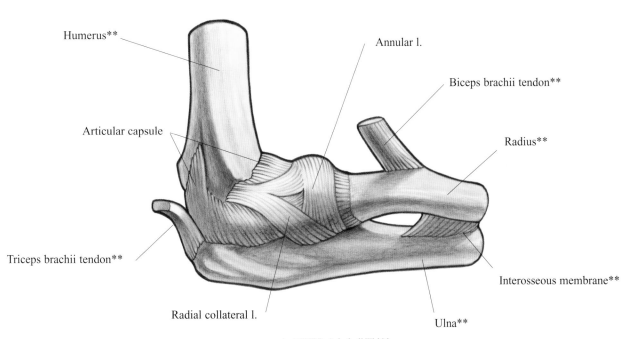

Humerus**

Annular l.

Biceps brachii tendon**

Articular capsule

Radius**

Triceps brachii tendon**

Interosseous membrane**

Radial collateral l.

Ulna**

LATERAL VIEW

JOINTS & LIGAMENTS

WRIST & HAND

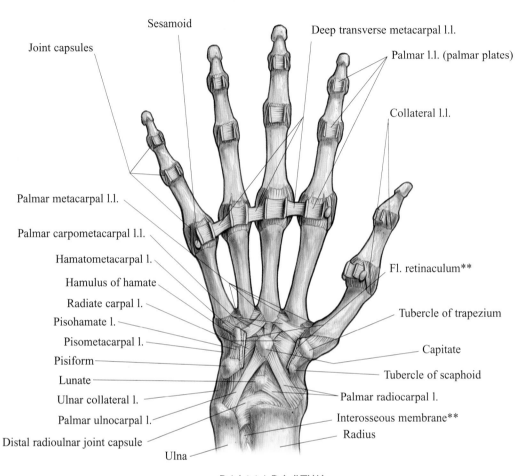

Sesamoid

Joint capsules

Deep transverse metacarpal l.l.

Palmar l.l. (palmar plates)

Collateral l.l.

Palmar metacarpal l.l.

Palmar carpometacarpal l.l.

Hamatometacarpal l.

Hamulus of hamate

Radiate carpal l.

Pisohamate l.

Pisometacarpal l.

Pisiform

Lunate

Ulnar collateral l.

Palmar ulnocarpal l.

Distal radioulnar joint capsule

Ulna

Fl. retinaculum**

Tubercle of trapezium

Capitate

Tubercle of scaphoid

Palmar radiocarpal l.

Interosseous membrane**

Radius

PALMAR VIEW

WRIST

FINGER

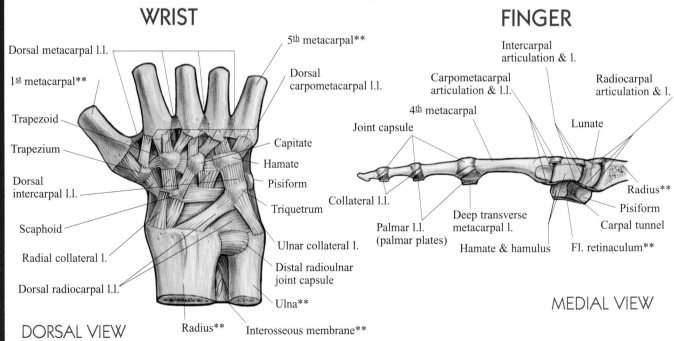

Dorsal metacarpal l.l.

1st metacarpal**

Trapezoid

Trapezium

Dorsal intercarpal l.l.

Scaphoid

Radial collateral l.

Dorsal radiocarpal l.l.

5th metacarpal**

Dorsal carpometacarpal l.l.

Capitate

Hamate

Pisiform

Triquetrum

Ulnar collateral l.

Distal radioulnar joint capsule

Ulna**

Radius**

Interosseous membrane**

Intercarpal articulation & l.

Carpometacarpal articulation & l.l.

4th metacarpal

Joint capsule

Collateral l.l.

Palmar l.l. (palmar plates)

Deep transverse metacarpal l.

Hamate & hamulus

Radiocarpal articulation & l.

Lunate

Radius**

Pisiform

Carpal tunnel

Fl. retinaculum**

DORSAL VIEW

MEDIAL VIEW

LUMBAR SPINE

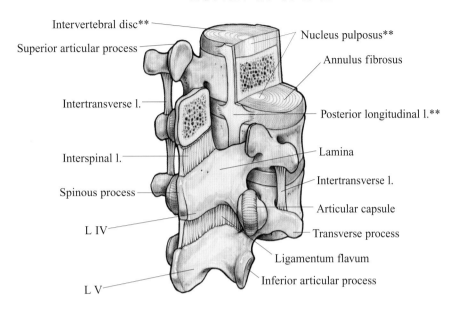

Intervertebral disc**

Superior articular process

Nucleus pulposus**

Annulus fibrosus

Intertransverse l.

Posterior longitudinal l.**

Interspinal l.

Lamina

Intertransverse l.

Spinous process

Articular capsule

L IV

Transverse process

Ligamentum flavum

Inferior articular process

L V

CONNECTIVE COMPONENTS OF THE PELVIS

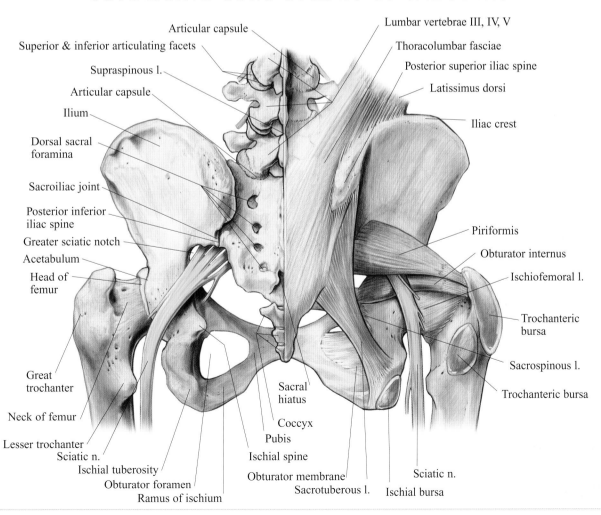

Articular capsule

Lumbar vertebrae III, IV, V

Superior & inferior articulating facets

Thoracolumbar fasciae

Supraspinous l.

Posterior superior iliac spine

Articular capsule

Latissimus dorsi

Ilium

Iliac crest

Dorsal sacral foramina

Sacroiliac joint

Posterior inferior iliac spine

Piriformis

Greater sciatic notch

Obturator internus

Acetabulum

Ischiofemoral l.

Head of femur

Trochanteric bursa

Great trochanter

Sacrospinous l.

Trochanteric bursa

Neck of femur

Sacral hiatus

Lesser trochanter

Coccyx

Sciatic n.

Pubis

Ischial tuberosity

Ischial spine

Obturator foramen

Obturator membrane

Sciatic n.

Ramus of ischium

Sacrotuberous l.

Ischial bursa

HIP LIGAMENTS

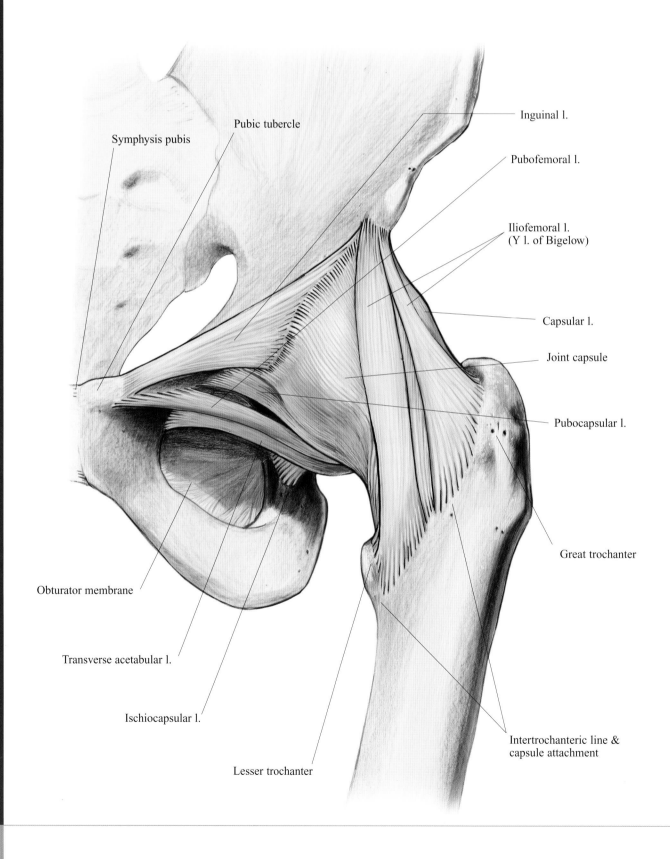

Symphysis pubis

Pubic tubercle

Inguinal l.

Pubofemoral l.

Iliofemoral l.
(Y l. of Bigelow)

Capsular l.

Joint capsule

Pubocapsular l.

Great trochanter

Obturator membrane

Transverse acetabular l.

Ischiocapsular l.

Intertrochanteric line &
capsule attachment

Lesser trochanter

HIP LIGAMENTS (OPENED)

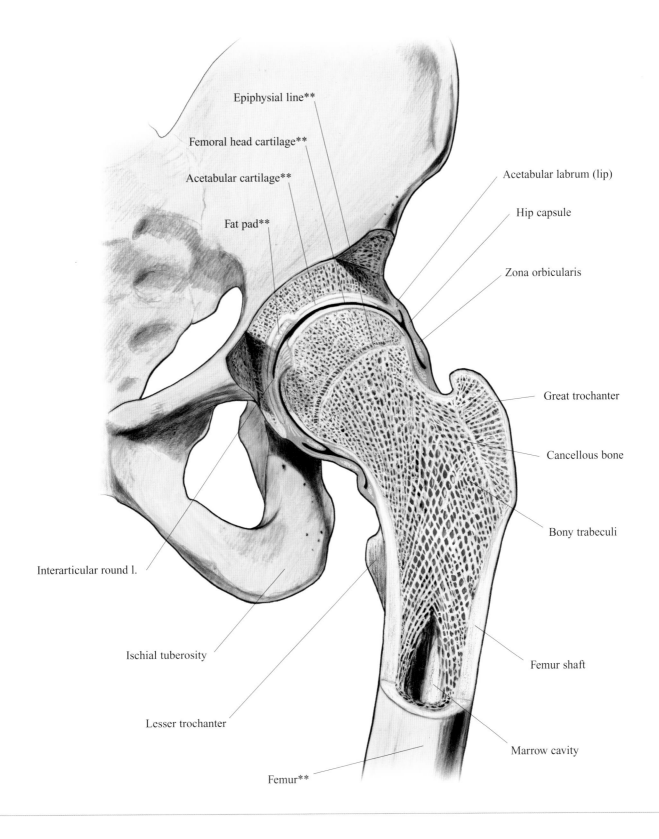

Epiphysial line**

Femoral head cartilage**

Acetabular cartilage**

Fat pad**

Acetabular labrum (lip)

Hip capsule

Zona orbicularis

Great trochanter

Cancellous bone

Bony trabeculi

Interarticular round l.

Ischial tuberosity

Lesser trochanter

Femur shaft

Marrow cavity

Femur**

JOINTS & LIGAMENTS

PELVIS

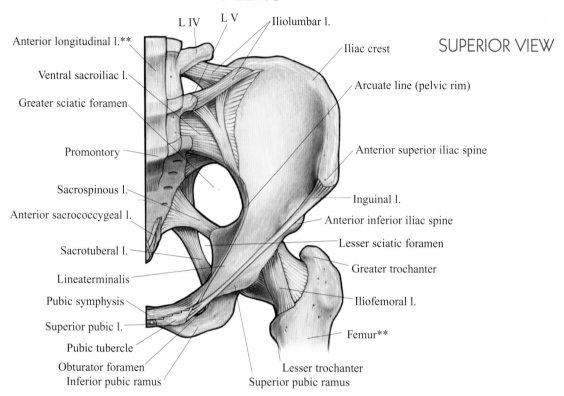

L IV   L V

SUPERIOR VIEW

- Anterior longitudinal l.**
- Ventral sacroiliac l.
- Greater sciatic foramen
- Promontory
- Sacrospinous l.
- Anterior sacrococcygeal l.
- Sacrotuberal l.
- Lineaterminalis
- Pubic symphysis
- Superior pubic l.
- Pubic tubercle
- Obturator foramen
- Inferior pubic ramus

- Iliolumbar l.
- Iliac crest
- Arcuate line (pelvic rim)
- Anterior superior iliac spine
- Inguinal l.
- Anterior inferior iliac spine
- Lesser sciatic foramen
- Greater trochanter
- Iliofemoral l.
- Femur**
- Lesser trochanter
- Superior pubic ramus

PELVIS

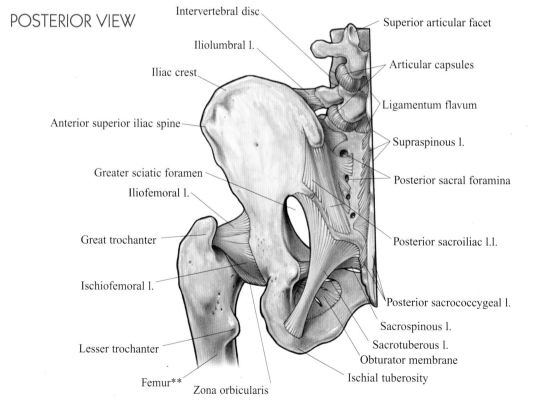

POSTERIOR VIEW

- Intervertebral disc
- Iliolumbral l.
- Iliac crest
- Anterior superior iliac spine
- Greater sciatic foramen
- Iliofemoral l.
- Great trochanter
- Ischiofemoral l.
- Lesser trochanter
- Femur**
- Zona orbicularis

- Superior articular facet
- Articular capsules
- Ligamentum flavum
- Supraspinous l.
- Posterior sacral foramina
- Posterior sacroiliac l.l.
- Posterior sacrococcygeal l.
- Sacrospinous l.
- Sacrotuberous l.
- Obturator membrane
- Ischial tuberosity

KNEE LIGAMENTS

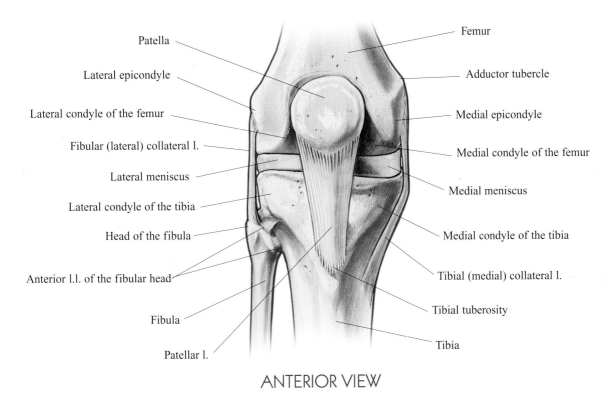

Patella

Lateral epicondyle

Lateral condyle of the femur

Fibular (lateral) collateral l.

Lateral meniscus

Lateral condyle of the tibia

Head of the fibula

Anterior l.l. of the fibular head

Fibula

Patellar l.

Femur

Adductor tubercle

Medial epicondyle

Medial condyle of the femur

Medial meniscus

Medial condyle of the tibia

Tibial (medial) collateral l.

Tibial tuberosity

Tibia

ANTERIOR VIEW

KNEE LIGAMENTS

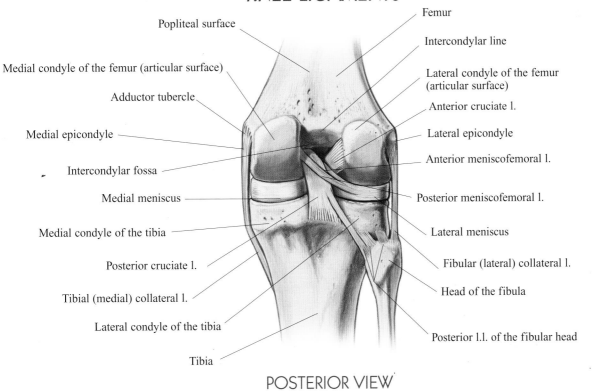

Popliteal surface

Medial condyle of the femur (articular surface)

Adductor tubercle

Medial epicondyle

Intercondylar fossa

Medial meniscus

Medial condyle of the tibia

Posterior cruciate l.

Tibial (medial) collateral l.

Lateral condyle of the tibia

Tibia

Femur

Intercondylar line

Lateral condyle of the femur (articular surface)

Anterior cruciate l.

Lateral epicondyle

Anterior meniscofemoral l.

Posterior meniscofemoral l.

Lateral meniscus

Fibular (lateral) collateral l.

Head of the fibula

Posterior l.l. of the fibular head

POSTERIOR VIEW

JOINTS & LIGAMENTS

RIGHT FOOT

LATERAL VIEW

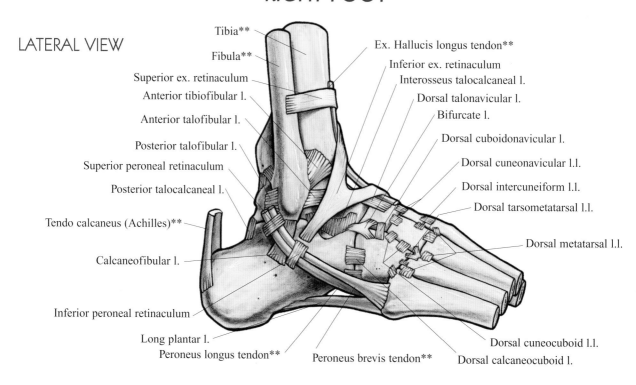

Tibia**
Fibula**
Superior ex. retinaculum
Anterior tibiofibular l.
Anterior talofibular l.
Posterior talofibular l.
Superior peroneal retinaculum
Posterior talocalcaneal l.
Tendo calcaneus (Achilles)**
Calcaneofibular l.
Inferior peroneal retinaculum
Long plantar l.
Peroneus longus tendon**
Peroneus brevis tendon**

Ex. Hallucis longus tendon**
Inferior ex. retinaculum
Interosseus talocalcaneal l.
Dorsal talonavicular l.
Bifurcate l.
Dorsal cuboidonavicular l.
Dorsal cuneonavicular l.l.
Dorsal intercuneiform l.l.
Dorsal tarsometatarsal l.l.
Dorsal metatarsal l.l.
Dorsal cuneocuboid l.l.
Dorsal calcaneocuboid l.

RIGHT FOOT

MEDIAL VIEW

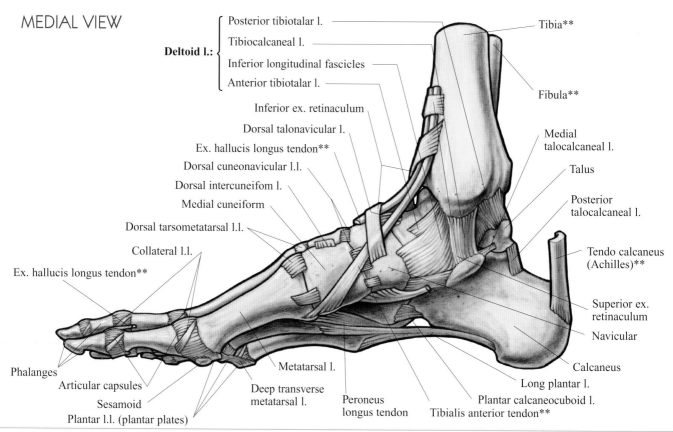

Deltoid l.: {
Posterior tibiotalar l.
Tibiocalcaneal l.
Inferior longitudinal fascicles
Anterior tibiotalar l.
}
Inferior ex. retinaculum
Dorsal talonavicular l.
Ex. hallucis longus tendon**
Dorsal cuneonavicular l.l.
Dorsal intercuneifom l.
Medial cuneiform
Dorsal tarsometatarsal l.l.
Collateral l.l.
Ex. hallucis longus tendon**
Phalanges
Articular capsules
Sesamoid
Plantar l.l. (plantar plates)
Metatarsal l.
Deep transverse metatarsal l.
Peroneus longus tendon
Tibialis anterior tendon**

Tibia**
Fibula**
Medial talocalcaneal l.
Talus
Posterior talocalcaneal l.
Tendo calcaneus (Achilles)**
Superior ex. retinaculum
Navicular
Calcaneus
Long plantar l.
Plantar calcaneocuboid l.

44

RIGHT FOOT

INFERIOR VIEW

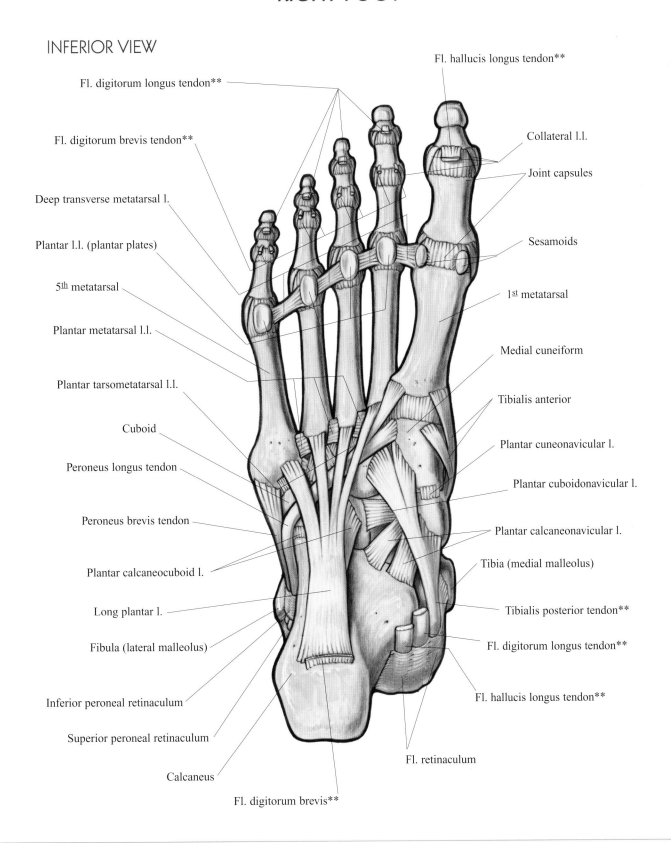

Fl. digitorum longus tendon**

Fl. digitorum brevis tendon**

Deep transverse metatarsal l.

Plantar l.l. (plantar plates)

5th metatarsal

Plantar metatarsal l.l.

Plantar tarsometatarsal l.l.

Cuboid

Peroneus longus tendon

Peroneus brevis tendon

Plantar calcaneocuboid l.

Long plantar l.

Fibula (lateral malleolus)

Inferior peroneal retinaculum

Superior peroneal retinaculum

Calcaneus

Fl. digitorum brevis**

Fl. hallucis longus tendon**

Collateral l.l.

Joint capsules

Sesamoids

1st metatarsal

Medial cuneiform

Tibialis anterior

Plantar cuneonavicular l.

Plantar cuboidonavicular l.

Plantar calcaneonavicular l.

Tibia (medial malleolus)

Tibialis posterior tendon**

Fl. digitorum longus tendon**

Fl. hallucis longus tendon**

Fl. retinaculum

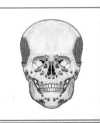

4

ORIGINS & INSERTIONS

HEAD & TRUNK

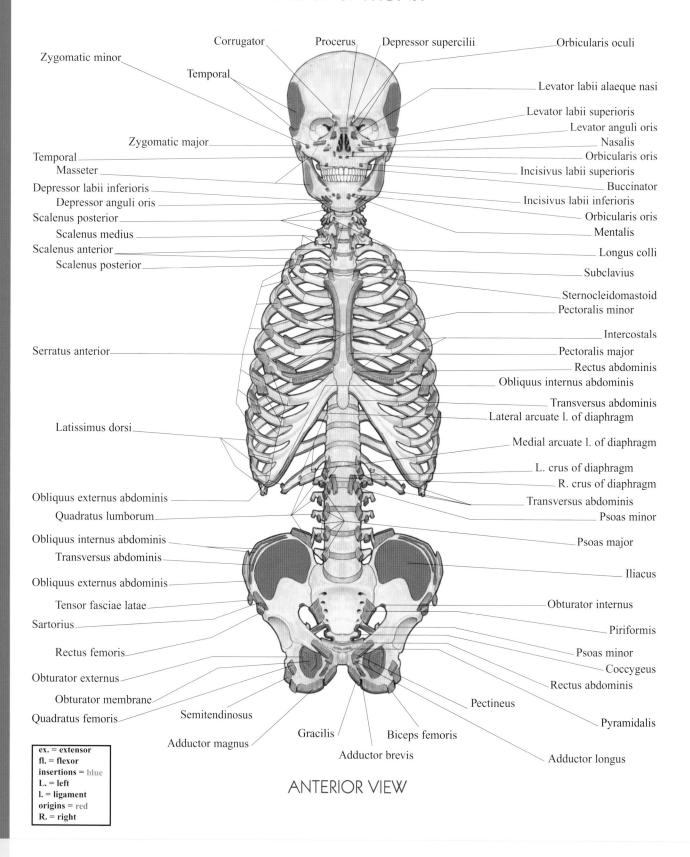

Corrugator Procerus Depressor supercilii Orbicularis oculi

Zygomatic minor

Temporal

Levator labii alaeque nasi

Levator labii superioris

Levator anguli oris

Zygomatic major

Nasalis

Temporal

Orbicularis oris

Masseter

Incisivus labii superioris

Depressor labii inferioris

Buccinator

Depressor anguli oris

Incisivus labii inferioris

Scalenus posterior

Orbicularis oris

Scalenus medius

Mentalis

Scalenus anterior

Longus colli

Scalenus posterior

Subclavius

Sternocleidomastoid

Pectoralis minor

Intercostals

Serratus anterior

Pectoralis major

Rectus abdominis

Obliquus internus abdominis

Transversus abdominis

Lateral arcuate l. of diaphragm

Latissimus dorsi

Medial arcuate l. of diaphragm

L. crus of diaphragm

R. crus of diaphragm

Transversus abdominis

Obliquus externus abdominis

Psoas minor

Quadratus lumborum

Obliquus internus abdominis

Psoas major

Transversus abdominis

Obliquus externus abdominis

Iliacus

Tensor fasciae latae

Obturator internus

Sartorius

Piriformis

Psoas minor

Rectus femoris

Coccygeus

Obturator externus

Rectus abdominis

Obturator membrane

Quadratus femoris

Pyramidalis

Semitendinosus

Pectineus

Adductor magnus Gracilis Biceps femoris

Adductor brevis

Adductor longus

ex. = extensor
fl. = flexor
insertions = blue
L. = left
l. = ligament
origins = red
R. = right

ANTERIOR VIEW

48

HEAD & TRUNK

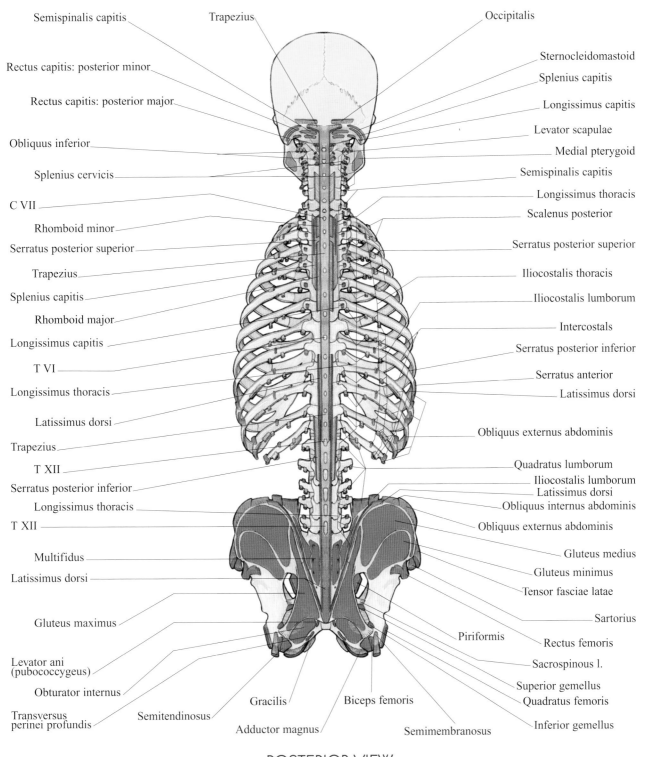

Semispinalis capitis

Rectus capitis: posterior minor

Rectus capitis: posterior major

Obliquus inferior

Splenius cervicis

C VII

Rhomboid minor

Serratus posterior superior

Trapezius

Splenius capitis

Rhomboid major

Longissimus capitis

T VI

Longissimus thoracis

Latissimus dorsi

Trapezius

T XII

Serratus posterior inferior

Longissimus thoracis

T XII

Multifidus

Latissimus dorsi

Gluteus maximus

Levator ani
(pubococcygeus)

Obturator internus

Transversus
perinei profundis

Trapezius

Semitendinosus

Gracilis

Adductor magnus

Biceps femoris

Semimembranosus

Occipitalis

Sternocleidomastoid

Splenius capitis

Longissimus capitis

Levator scapulae

Medial pterygoid

Semispinalis capitis

Longissimus thoracis

Scalenus posterior

Serratus posterior superior

Iliocostalis thoracis

Iliocostalis lumborum

Intercostals

Serratus posterior inferior

Serratus anterior

Latissimus dorsi

Obliquus externus abdominis

Quadratus lumborum

Iliocostalis lumborum

Latissimus dorsi

Obliquus internus abdominis

Obliquus externus abdominis

Gluteus medius

Gluteus minimus

Tensor fasciae latae

Sartorius

Piriformis

Rectus femoris

Sacrospinous l.

Superior gemellus

Quadratus femoris

Inferior gemellus

POSTERIOR VIEW

ARM

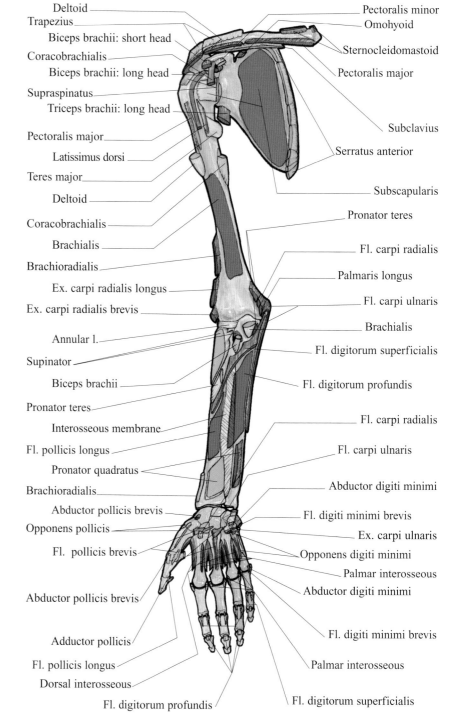

Deltoid
Trapezius
Biceps brachii: short head
Coracobrachialis
Biceps brachii: long head
Supraspinatus
Triceps brachii: long head
Pectoralis major
Latissimus dorsi
Teres major
Deltoid
Coracobrachialis
Brachialis
Brachioradialis
Ex. carpi radialis longus
Ex. carpi radialis brevis
Annular l.
Supinator
Biceps brachii
Pronator teres
Interosseous membrane
Fl. pollicis longus
Pronator quadratus
Brachioradialis
Abductor pollicis brevis
Opponens pollicis
Fl. pollicis brevis
Abductor pollicis brevis
Adductor pollicis
Fl. pollicis longus
Dorsal interosseous
Fl. digitorum profundis

Pectoralis minor
Omohyoid
Sternocleidomastoid
Pectoralis major
Subclavius
Serratus anterior
Subscapularis
Pronator teres
Fl. carpi radialis
Palmaris longus
Fl. carpi ulnaris
Brachialis
Fl. digitorum superficialis
Fl. digitorum profundis
Fl. carpi radialis
Fl. carpi ulnaris
Abductor digiti minimi
Fl. digiti minimi brevis
Ex. carpi ulnaris
Opponens digiti minimi
Palmar interosseous
Abductor digiti minimi
Fl. digiti minimi brevis
Palmar interosseous
Fl. digitorum superficialis

ANTERIOR VIEW

CLAVICLE
SUPERIOR VIEW

ANTERIOR

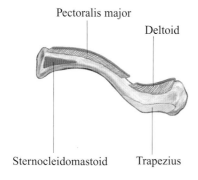

Pectoralis major
Deltoid
Sternocleidomastoid
Trapezius

POSTERIOR

ARM

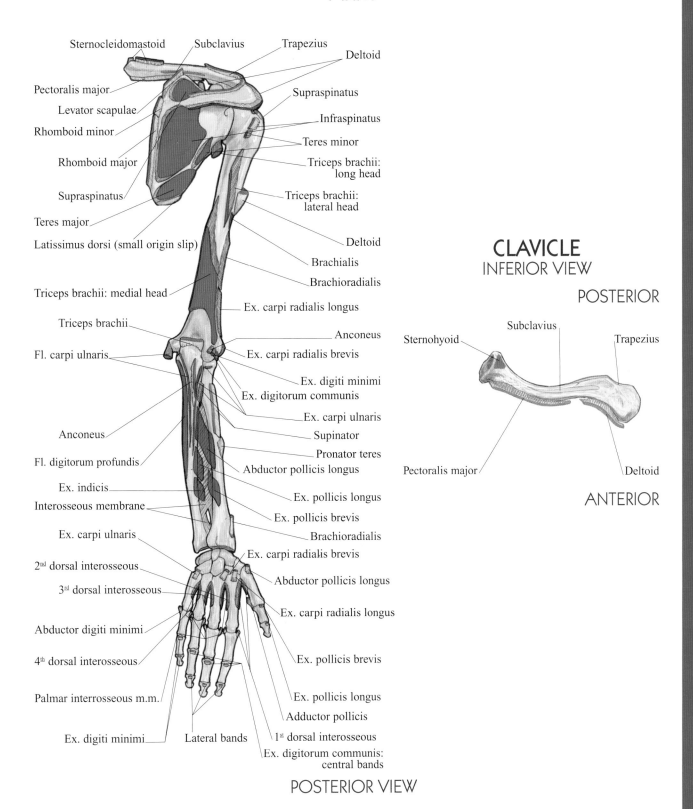

Sternocleidomastoid

Subclavius

Trapezius

Deltoid

Pectoralis major

Levator scapulae

Rhomboid minor

Rhomboid major

Supraspinatus

Teres major

Latissimus dorsi (small origin slip)

Triceps brachii: medial head

Triceps brachii

Fl. carpi ulnaris

Anconeus

Fl. digitorum profundis

Ex. indicis

Interosseous membrane

Ex. carpi ulnaris

2nd dorsal interosseous

3rd dorsal interosseous

Abductor digiti minimi

4th dorsal interosseous

Palmar interrosseous m.m.

Ex. digiti minimi

Supraspinatus

Infraspinatus

Teres minor

Triceps brachii: long head

Triceps brachii: lateral head

Deltoid

Brachialis

Brachioradialis

Ex. carpi radialis longus

Anconeus

Ex. carpi radialis brevis

Ex. digiti minimi

Ex. digitorum communis

Ex. carpi ulnaris

Supinator

Pronator teres

Abductor pollicis longus

Ex. pollicis longus

Ex. pollicis brevis

Brachioradialis

Ex. carpi radialis brevis

Abductor pollicis longus

Ex. carpi radialis longus

Ex. pollicis brevis

Ex. pollicis longus

Adductor pollicis

1st dorsal interosseous

Ex. digitorum communis: central bands

Lateral bands

POSTERIOR VIEW

CLAVICLE
INFERIOR VIEW

POSTERIOR

Sternohyoid

Subclavius

Trapezius

Pectoralis major

Deltoid

ANTERIOR

HAND

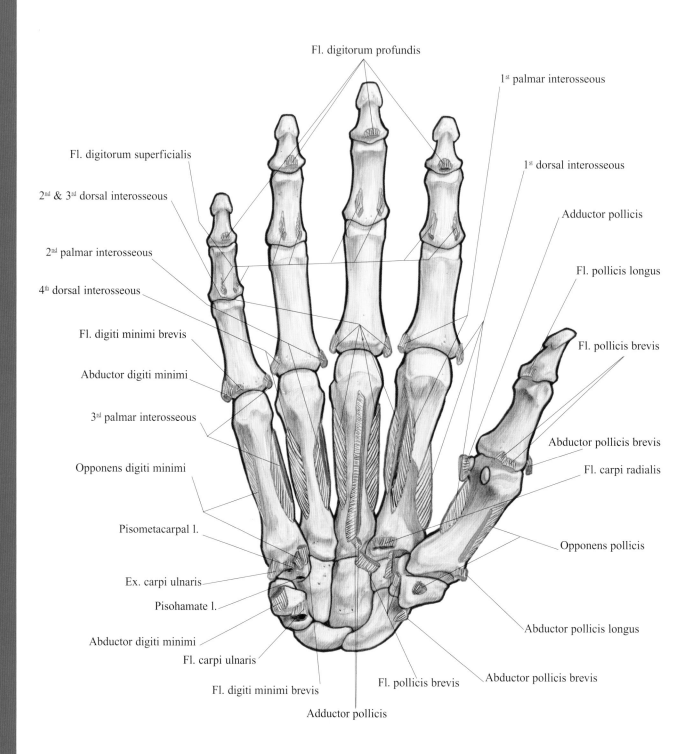

Fl. digitorum profundis

1ˢᵗ palmar interosseous

Fl. digitorum superficialis

1ˢᵗ dorsal interosseous

2ⁿᵈ & 3ʳᵈ dorsal interosseous

Adductor pollicis

2ⁿᵈ palmar interosseous

Fl. pollicis longus

4ᵗʰ dorsal interosseous

Fl. digiti minimi brevis

Fl. pollicis brevis

Abductor digiti minimi

3ʳᵈ palmar interosseous

Abductor pollicis brevis

Fl. carpi radialis

Opponens digiti minimi

Pisometacarpal l.

Opponens pollicis

Ex. carpi ulnaris

Pisohamate l.

Abductor digiti minimi

Abductor pollicis longus

Fl. carpi ulnaris

Fl. digiti minimi brevis

Fl. pollicis brevis

Abductor pollicis brevis

Adductor pollicis

PALMAR VIEW

HAND

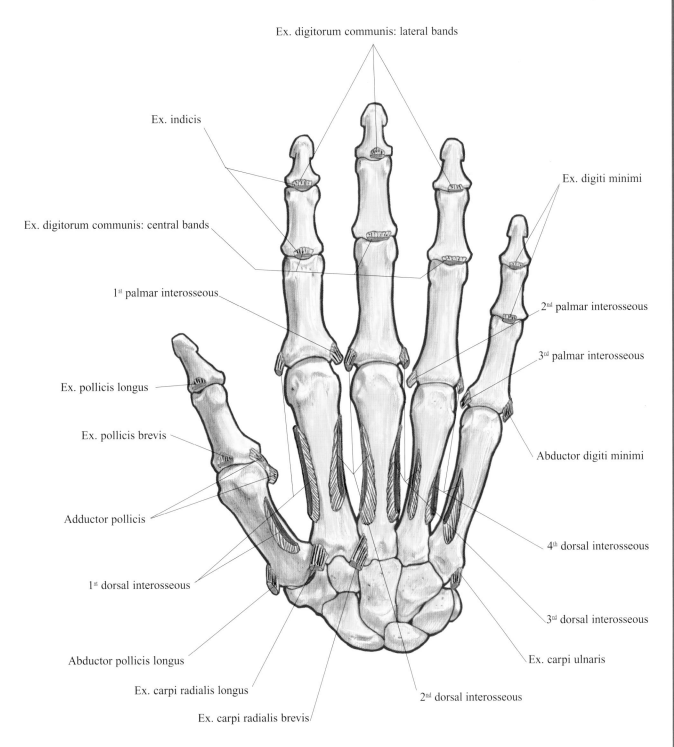

Ex. digitorum communis: lateral bands

Ex. indicis

Ex. digitorum communis: central bands

1ˢᵗ palmar interosseous

Ex. pollicis longus

Ex. pollicis brevis

Adductor pollicis

1ˢᵗ dorsal interosseous

Abductor pollicis longus

Ex. carpi radialis longus

Ex. carpi radialis brevis

Ex. digiti minimi

2ⁿᵈ palmar interosseous

3ʳᵈ palmar interosseous

Abductor digiti minimi

4ᵗʰ dorsal interosseous

3ʳᵈ dorsal interosseous

Ex. carpi ulnaris

2ⁿᵈ dorsal interosseous

DORSAL VIEW

LEG & FOOT

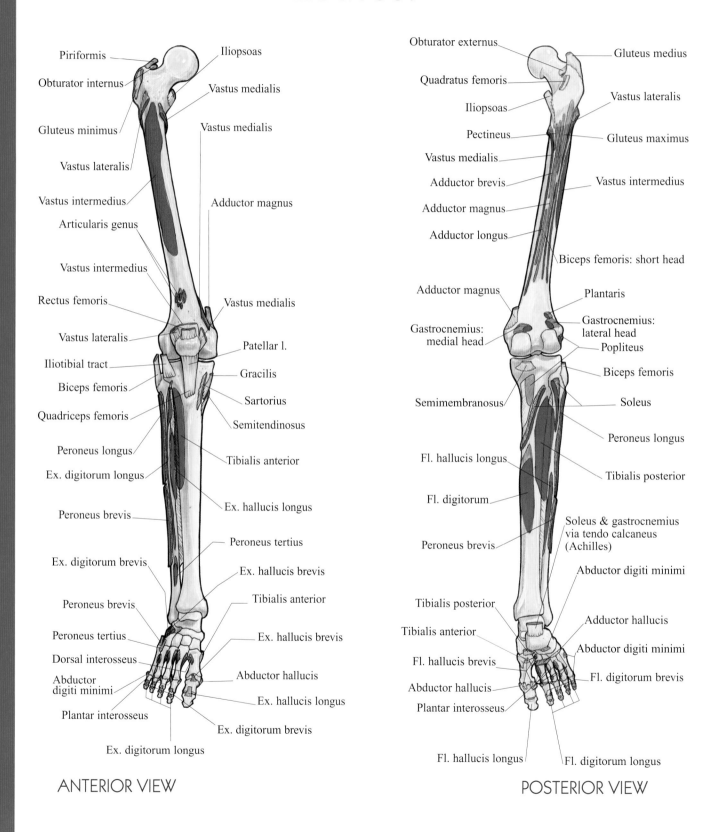

ANTERIOR VIEW

Piriformis
Obturator internus
Gluteus minimus
Vastus lateralis
Vastus intermedius
Articularis genus
Vastus intermedius
Rectus femoris
Vastus lateralis
Iliotibial tract
Biceps femoris
Quadriceps femoris
Peroneus longus
Ex. digitorum longus
Peroneus brevis
Ex. digitorum brevis
Peroneus brevis
Peroneus tertius
Dorsal interosseus
Abductor digiti minimi
Plantar interosseus
Ex. digitorum longus

Iliopsoas
Vastus medialis
Vastus medialis
Adductor magnus
Vastus medialis
Patellar l.
Gracilis
Sartorius
Semitendinosus
Tibialis anterior
Ex. hallucis longus
Peroneus tertius
Ex. hallucis brevis
Tibialis anterior
Ex. hallucis brevis
Abductor hallucis
Ex. hallucis longus
Ex. digitorum brevis

POSTERIOR VIEW

Obturator externus
Quadratus femoris
Iliopsoas
Pectineus
Vastus medialis
Adductor brevis
Adductor magnus
Adductor longus
Adductor magnus
Gastrocnemius: medial head
Semimembranosus
Fl. hallucis longus
Fl. digitorum
Peroneus brevis
Tibialis posterior
Tibialis anterior
Fl. hallucis brevis
Abductor hallucis
Plantar interosseus
Fl. hallucis longus

Gluteus medius
Vastus lateralis
Gluteus maximus
Vastus intermedius
Biceps femoris: short head
Plantaris
Gastrocnemius: lateral head
Popliteus
Biceps femoris
Soleus
Peroneus longus
Tibialis posterior
Soleus & gastrocnemius via tendo calcaneus (Achilles)
Abductor digiti minimi
Adductor hallucis
Abductor digiti minimi
Fl. digitorum brevis
Fl. digitorum longus

FOOT

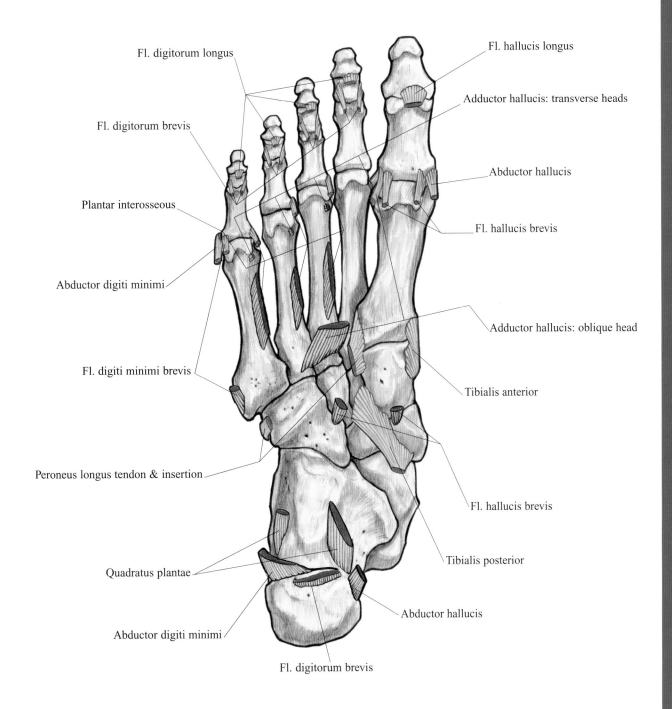

Fl. digitorum longus

Fl. digitorum brevis

Plantar interosseous

Abductor digiti minimi

Fl. digiti minimi brevis

Peroneus longus tendon & insertion

Quadratus plantae

Abductor digiti minimi

Fl. digitorum brevis

Fl. hallucis longus

Adductor hallucis: transverse heads

Abductor hallucis

Fl. hallucis brevis

Adductor hallucis: oblique head

Tibialis anterior

Fl. hallucis brevis

Tibialis posterior

Abductor hallucis

PLANTAR VIEW

FOOT

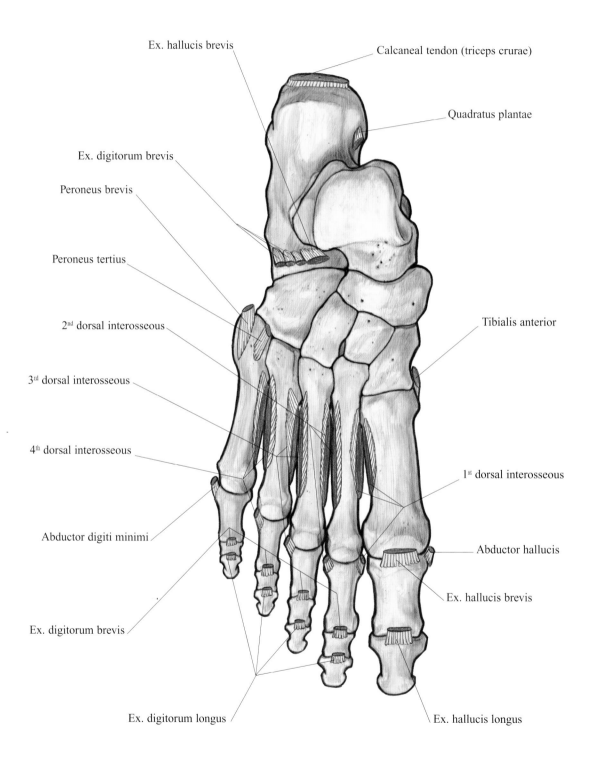

Ex. hallucis brevis

Calcaneal tendon (triceps crurae)

Ex. digitorum brevis

Quadratus plantae

Peroneus brevis

Peroneus tertius

2nd dorsal interosseous

3rd dorsal interosseous

Tibialis anterior

4th dorsal interosseous

1st dorsal interosseous

Abductor digiti minimi

Abductor hallucis

Ex. hallucis brevis

Ex. digitorum brevis

Ex. digitorum longus

Ex. hallucis longus

DORSAL VIEW

BASE OF SKULL

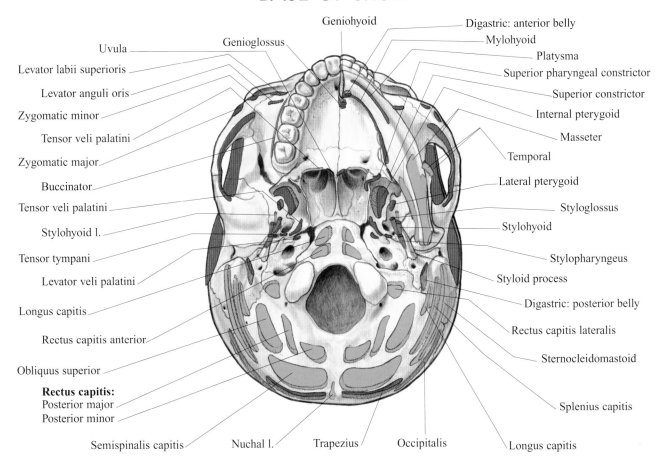

Geniohyoid
Genioglossus
Uvula
Levator labii superioris
Levator anguli oris
Zygomatic minor
Tensor veli palatini
Zygomatic major
Buccinator
Tensor veli palatini
Stylohyoid l.
Tensor tympani
Levator veli palatini
Longus capitis
Rectus capitis anterior
Obliquus superior
Rectus capitis:
Posterior major
Posterior minor
Semispinalis capitis
Nuchal l.
Trapezius
Occipitalis

Digastric: anterior belly
Mylohyoid
Platysma
Superior pharyngeal constrictor
Superior constrictor
Internal pterygoid
Masseter
Temporal
Lateral pterygoid
Styloglossus
Stylohyoid
Stylopharyngeus
Styloid process
Digastric: posterior belly
Rectus capitis lateralis
Sternocleidomastoid
Splenius capitis
Longus capitis

HYOID BONE

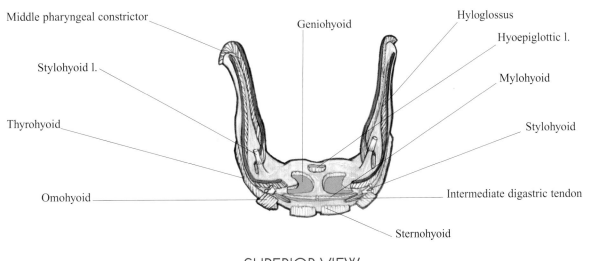

Middle pharyngeal constrictor
Stylohyoid l.
Thyrohyoid
Omohyoid

Geniohyoid

Hyloglossus
Hyoepiglottic l.
Mylohyoid
Stylohyoid
Intermediate digastric tendon

Sternohyoid

SUPERIOR VIEW

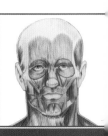

5

MUSCULAR SYSTEM

MUSCULAR SYSTEM

SURFACE MUSCLES

LAYER I

LAYER II

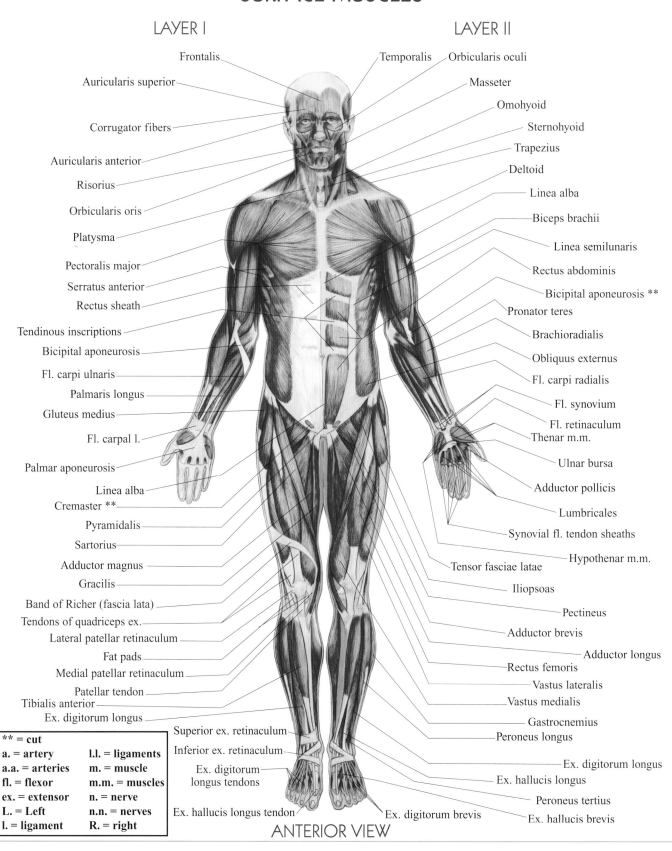

Frontalis

Auricularis superior

Corrugator fibers

Auricularis anterior

Risorius

Orbicularis oris

Platysma

Pectoralis major

Serratus anterior

Rectus sheath

Tendinous inscriptions

Bicipital aponeurosis

Fl. carpi ulnaris

Palmaris longus

Gluteus medius

Fl. carpal l.

Palmar aponeurosis

Linea alba

Cremaster **

Pyramidalis

Sartorius

Adductor magnus

Gracilis

Band of Richer (fascia lata)

Tendons of quadriceps ex.

Lateral patellar retinaculum

Fat pads

Medial patellar retinaculum

Patellar tendon

Tibialis anterior

Ex. digitorum longus

Temporalis

Orbicularis oculi

Masseter

Omohyoid

Sternohyoid

Trapezius

Deltoid

Linea alba

Biceps brachii

Linea semilunaris

Rectus abdominis

Bicipital aponeurosis **

Pronator teres

Brachioradialis

Obliquus externus

Fl. carpi radialis

Fl. synovium

Fl. retinaculum

Thenar m.m.

Ulnar bursa

Adductor pollicis

Lumbricales

Synovial fl. tendon sheaths

Hypothenar m.m.

Tensor fasciae latae

Iliopsoas

Pectineus

Adductor brevis

Adductor longus

Rectus femoris

Vastus lateralis

Vastus medialis

Gastrocnemius

Peroneus longus

Ex. digitorum longus

Ex. hallucis longus

Peroneus tertius

Ex. hallucis brevis

Superior ex. retinaculum

Inferior ex. retinaculum

Ex. digitorum longus tendons

Ex. hallucis longus tendon

Ex. digitorum brevis

ANTERIOR VIEW

** = cut	
a. = artery	l.l. = ligaments
a.a. = arteries	m. = muscle
fl. = flexor	m.m. = muscles
ex. = extensor	n. = nerve
L. = Left	n.n. = nerves
l. = ligament	R. = right

DEEP MUSCLES

LAYER III

LAYER IV

Corrugator supercilii
Temporalis
Levator labii superioris
Zygomatic minor
Levator labii alaeque nasi
Buccinator
Masseter
Depressor labii inferioris
Omohyoid: superior belly
Subclavius
Supraspinatus
Omohyoid: inferior belly
Subscapularis
Sternohyoid
Pectoralis minor
Biceps brachii: short head
Biceps brachii: long head
Internal intercostals
Supinator
Fl. pollicis longus
Adductor pollicis
Lumbricales
Fl. retinaculum
Fl. carpi ulnaris**
Annular l.
Fl. digitorum superficialis
Gluteus minimus
Obliquus internus
Iliopsoas
Pectineus
Iliotibial band**
Soleus
Ex. digitorum longus
Peroneus brevis
Peroneus tertius**
Ex. digitorum brevis
Ex. hallucis brevis
Adductor hallucis

Nasalis

Lateral nasal cartilage
Greater alar cartilage
Levator anguli oris
Incisivus labii superioris
Incisivus labii inferioris
Mentalis
Thyrohyoid
Scalenus medius
Scalenus anterior
Biceps brachii: long head**
Scalenus posterior
Latissimus dorsi
Lung
Coracobrachialis
Sternothyroid
Serratus anterior (9 slips)
Brachialis
Transversus thoracis
Fl. digitorum profundis
Innermost intercostals
Transversus abdominis
Linea alba
Arcuate line
Obturator externus
Adductor brevis
Adductor longus**
Adductor magnus
Vastus intermedius
Soleus
Gastrocnemius: medial head
Peroneus brevis
Ex. hallucis longus
Dorsal interosseous
Abductor hallucis

ANTERIOR VIEW

MUSCULAR SYSTEM

DEEP MUSCLES

LAYER V   LAYER VI

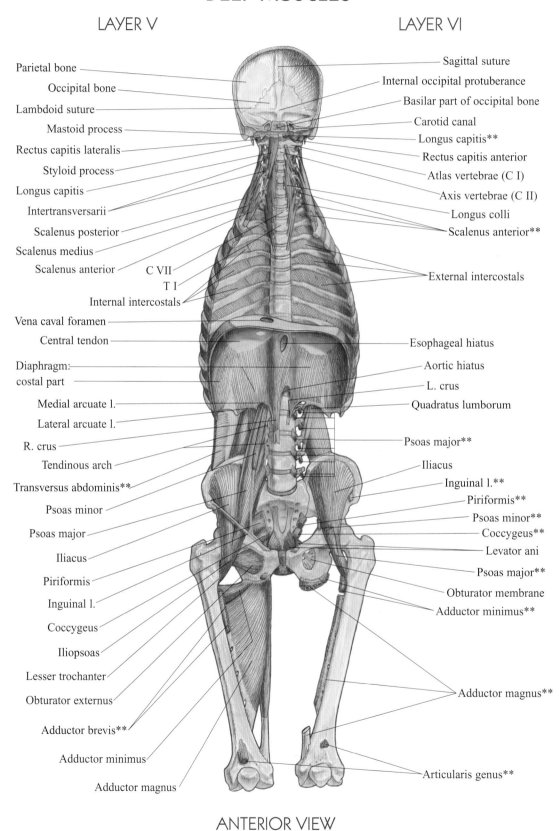

Parietal bone —
Occipital bone —
Lambdoid suture —
Mastoid process —
Rectus capitis lateralis —
Styloid process —
Longus capitis —
Intertransversarii —
Scalenus posterior —
Scalenus medius —
Scalenus anterior —   C VII
                        T I
Internal intercostals —
Vena caval foramen —
Central tendon —
Diaphragm: —
costal part —
Medial arcuate l. —
Lateral arcuate l. —
R. crus —
Tendinous arch —
Transversus abdominis** —
Psoas minor —
Psoas major —
Iliacus —
Piriformis —
Inguinal l. —
Coccygeus —
Iliopsoas —
Lesser trochanter —
Obturator externus —
Adductor brevis** —
Adductor minimus —
Adductor magnus —

Sagittal suture
Internal occipital protuberance
Basilar part of occipital bone
Carotid canal
Longus capitis**
Rectus capitis anterior
Atlas vertebrae (C I)
Axis vertebrae (C II)
Longus colli
Scalenus anterior**
External intercostals
Esophageal hiatus
Aortic hiatus
L. crus
Quadratus lumborum
Psoas major**
Iliacus
Inguinal l.**
Piriformis**
Psoas minor**
Coccygeus**
Levator ani
Psoas major**
Obturator membrane
Adductor minimus**
Adductor magnus**
Articularis genus**

ANTERIOR VIEW

SURFACE MUSCLES

LAYER I

Semispinalis capitis

Splenius capitis

Levator scapulae

Trapezius

Rhomboideus major

Teres major

Latissimus dorsi

Ex. carpi radialis longus

Anconeus

Ex. digitorum communis

Ex. carpi radialis brevis

Ex. carpi ulnaris
Abductor pollicis longus
Ex. pollicis brevis

Fl. carpi ulnaris

Adductor magnus

Vastus lateralis

Gracilis

Semitendinosus

Semimembranosus

Popliteal fossa

Inner hamstring tendons

Peroneus longus tendon

Tendo calcaneus (Achilles)

Fl. retinaculum

Occipitalis

Splenius capitis

Sternocleidomastoid

Deltoid

Infraspinatus

Teres minor

Triceps brachii

Ex. retinaculum

Gluteus medius

Gluteus maximus

Biceps femoris

Gastrocnemius

Soleus

Fl. digitorum longus

Peroneal retinaculum

Abductor hallucis

Fl. digitorum brevis

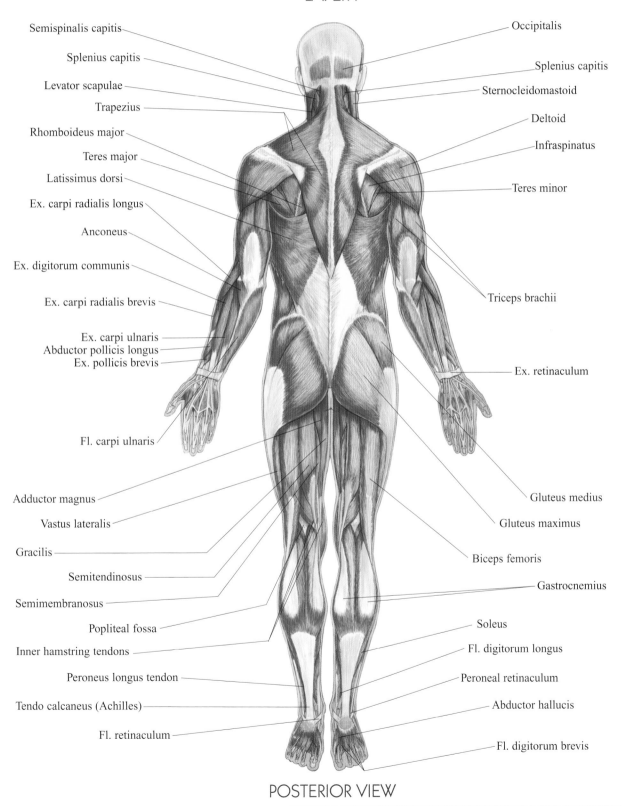

POSTERIOR VIEW

DEEP MUSCLES

LAYER II

LAYER III

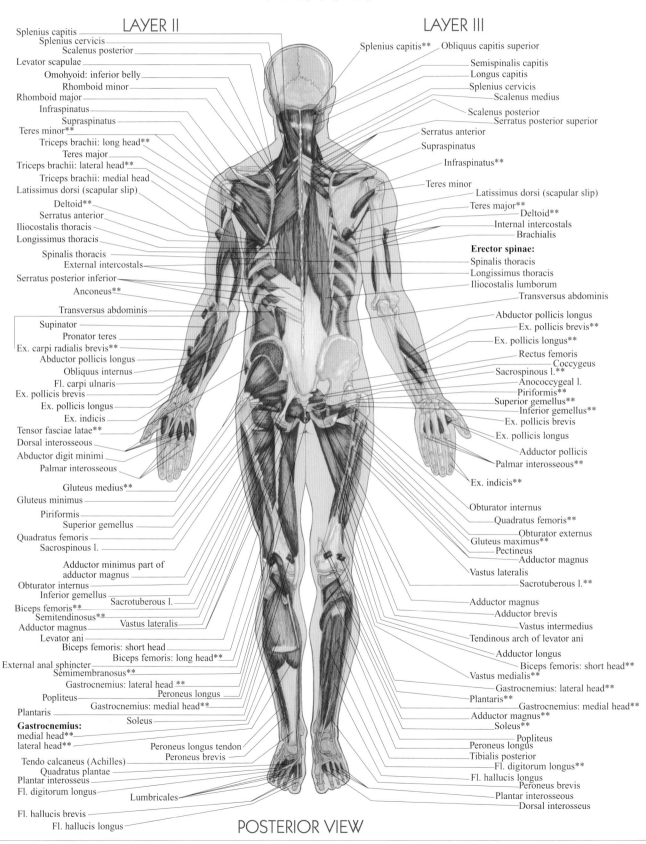

Splenius capitis
Splenius cervicis
Scalenus posterior
Levator scapulae
Omohyoid: inferior belly
Rhomboid minor
Rhomboid major
Infraspinatus
Supraspinatus
Teres minor**
Triceps brachii: long head**
Teres major
Triceps brachii: lateral head**
Triceps brachii: medial head
Latissimus dorsi (scapular slip)
Deltoid**
Serratus anterior
Iliocostalis thoracis
Longissimus thoracis
Spinalis thoracis
External intercostals
Serratus posterior inferior
Anconeus**
Transversus abdominis
Supinator
Pronator teres
Ex. carpi radialis brevis**
Abductor pollicis longus
Obliquus internus
Fl. carpi ulnaris
Ex. pollicis brevis
Ex. pollicis longus
Ex. indicis
Tensor fasciae latae**
Dorsal interosseous
Abductor digit minimi
Palmar interosseous
Gluteus medius**
Gluteus minimus
Piriformis
Superior gemellus
Quadratus femoris
Sacrospinous l.
Adductor minimus part of adductor magnus
Obturator internus
Inferior gemellus
Biceps femoris**
Semitendinosus**
Adductor magnus
Levator ani
Biceps femoris: short head
External anal sphincter
Semimembranosus**
Gastrocnemius: lateral head **
Popliteus
Plantaris
Gastrocnemius:
medial head**
lateral head**
Tendo calcaneus (Achilles)
Quadratus plantae
Plantar interosseus
Fl. digitorum longus
Fl. hallucis brevis
Fl. hallucis longus

Sacrotuberous l.
Vastus lateralis
Biceps femoris: long head**
Peroneus longus
Gastrocnemius: medial head**
Soleus
Peroneus longus tendon
Peroneus brevis
Lumbricales

Splenius capitis**
Obliquus capitis superior
Semispinalis capitis
Longus capitis
Splenius cervicis
Scalenus medius
Scalenus posterior
Serratus posterior superior
Serratus anterior
Supraspinatus
Infraspinatus**
Teres minor
Latissimus dorsi (scapular slip)
Teres major**
Deltoid**
Internal intercostals
Brachialis
Erector spinae:
Spinalis thoracis
Longissimus thoracis
Iliocostalis lumborum
Transversus abdominis
Abductor pollicis longus
Ex. pollicis brevis**
Ex. pollicis longus**
Rectus femoris
Coccygeus
Sacrospinous l.**
Anococcygeal l.
Piriformis**
Superior gemellus**
Inferior gemellus**
Ex. pollicis brevis
Ex. pollicis longus
Adductor pollicis
Palmar interosseous**
Ex. indicis**
Obturator internus
Quadratus femoris**
Obturator externus
Gluteus maximus**
Pectineus
Adductor magnus
Sacrotuberous l.**
Adductor magnus
Adductor brevis
Vastus intermedius
Tendinous arch of levator ani
Adductor longus
Biceps femoris: short head**
Vastus medialis**
Gastrocnemius: lateral head**
Plantaris**
Gastrocnemius: medial head**
Adductor magnus**
Soleus**
Popliteus
Peroneus longus
Tibialis posterior
Fl. digitorum longus**
Fl. hallucis longus
Peroneus brevis
Plantar interosseous
Dorsal interosseus

POSTERIOR VIEW

DEEP MUSCLES

LAYER IV

LAYER V

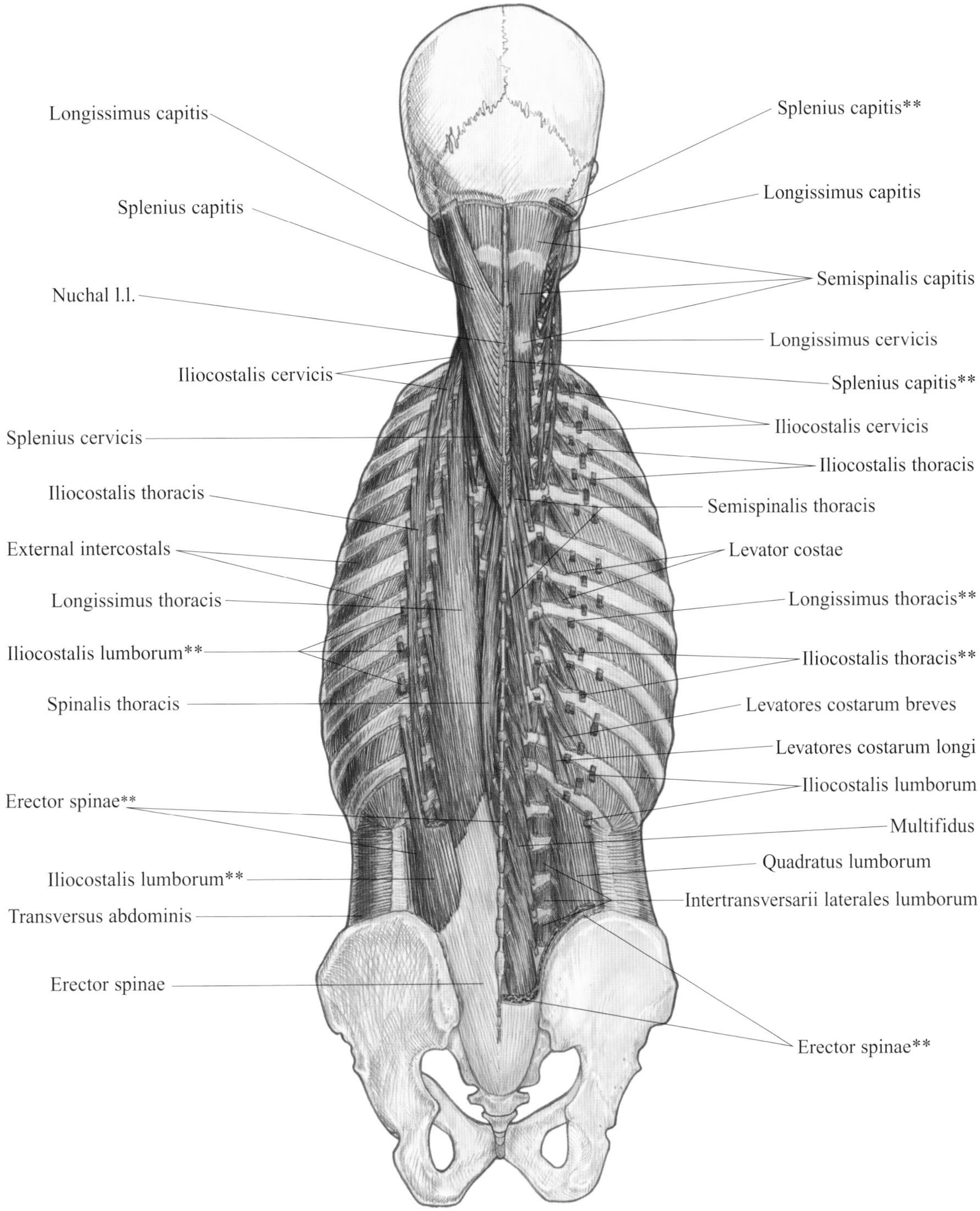

Longissimus capitis

Splenius capitis

Nuchal l.l.

Iliocostalis cervicis

Splenius cervicis

Iliocostalis thoracis

External intercostals

Longissimus thoracis

Iliocostalis lumborum**

Spinalis thoracis

Erector spinae**

Iliocostalis lumborum**

Transversus abdominis

Erector spinae

Splenius capitis**

Longissimus capitis

Semispinalis capitis

Longissimus cervicis

Splenius capitis**

Iliocostalis cervicis

Iliocostalis thoracis

Semispinalis thoracis

Levator costae

Longissimus thoracis**

Iliocostalis thoracis**

Levatores costarum breves

Levatores costarum longi

Iliocostalis lumborum

Multifidus

Quadratus lumborum

Intertransversarii laterales lumborum

Erector spinae**

POSTERIOR VIEW

DEEP MUSCLES

LAYER VI

LAYER VII

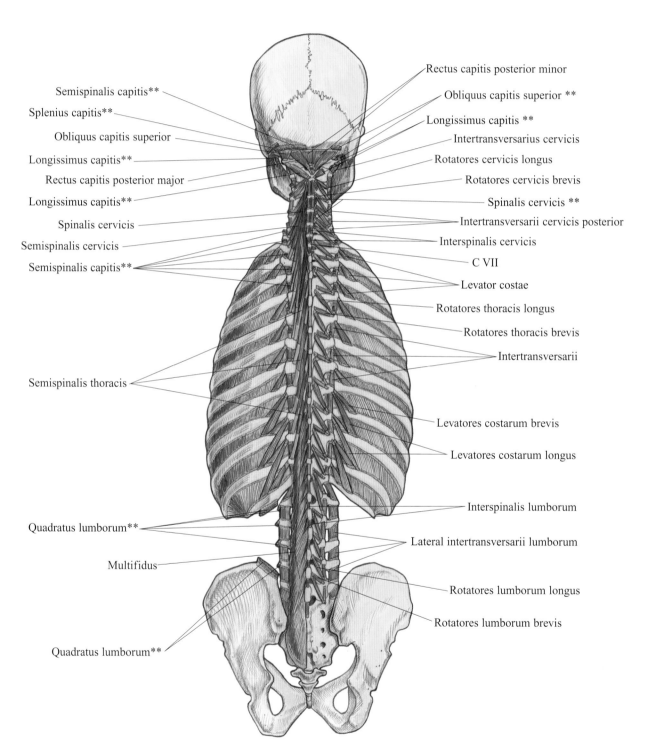

Semispinalis capitis**

Splenius capitis**

Obliquus capitis superior

Longissimus capitis**

Rectus capitis posterior major

Longissimus capitis**

Spinalis cervicis

Semispinalis cervicis

Semispinalis capitis**

Semispinalis thoracis

Quadratus lumborum**

Multifidus

Quadratus lumborum**

Rectus capitis posterior minor

Obliquus capitis superior **

Longissimus capitis **

Intertransversarius cervicis

Rotatores cervicis longus

Rotatores cervicis brevis

Spinalis cervicis **

Intertransversarii cervicis posterior

Interspinalis cervicis

C VII

Levator costae

Rotatores thoracis longus

Rotatores thoracis brevis

Intertransversarii

Levatores costarum brevis

Levatores costarum longus

Interspinalis lumborum

Lateral intertransversarii lumborum

Rotatores lumborum longus

Rotatores lumborum brevis

POSTERIOR VIEW

SURFACE MUSCLES

LAYER I

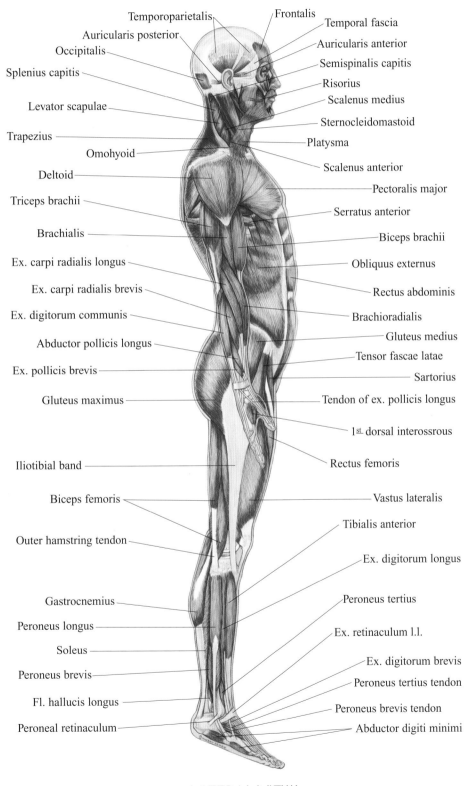

Temporoparietalis
Frontalis
Temporal fascia
Auricularis posterior
Auricularis anterior
Occipitalis
Semispinalis capitis
Splenius capitis
Risorius
Scalenus medius
Levator scapulae
Sternocleidomastoid
Trapezius
Platysma
Omohyoid
Scalenus anterior
Deltoid
Pectoralis major
Triceps brachii
Serratus anterior
Brachialis
Biceps brachii
Ex. carpi radialis longus
Obliquus externus
Ex. carpi radialis brevis
Rectus abdominis
Ex. digitorum communis
Brachioradialis
Abductor pollicis longus
Gluteus medius
Ex. pollicis brevis
Tensor fascae latae
Sartorius
Gluteus maximus
Tendon of ex. pollicis longus
1st dorsal interossrous
Rectus femoris
Iliotibial band
Biceps femoris
Vastus lateralis
Tibialis anterior
Outer hamstring tendon
Ex. digitorum longus
Gastrocnemius
Peroneus tertius
Peroneus longus
Ex. retinaculum l.l.
Soleus
Ex. digitorum brevis
Peroneus brevis
Peroneus tertius tendon
Fl. hallucis longus
Peroneus brevis tendon
Peroneal retinaculum
Abductor digiti minimi

LATERAL VIEW

SURFACE MUSCLES
LAYER IA

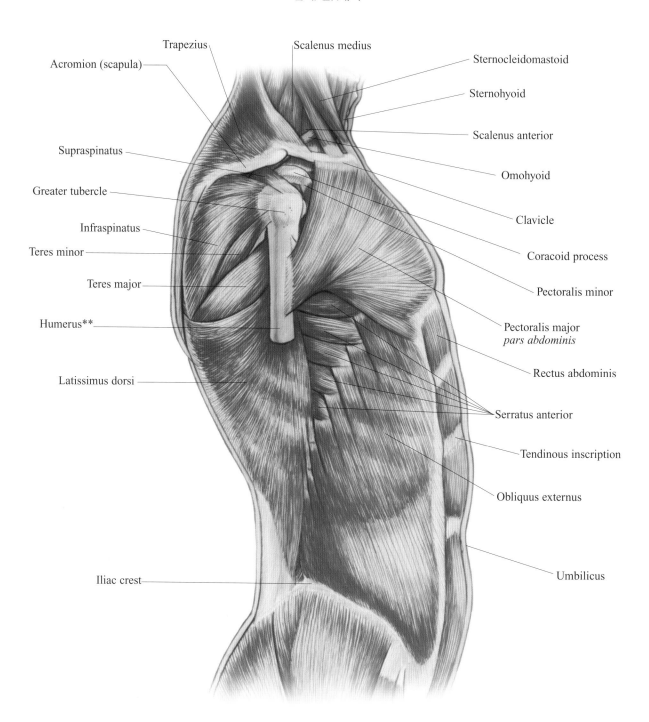

Trapezius

Scalenus medius

Sternocleidomastoid

Acromion (scapula)

Sternohyoid

Scalenus anterior

Supraspinatus

Omohyoid

Greater tubercle

Clavicle

Infraspinatus

Coracoid process

Teres minor

Pectoralis minor

Teres major

Pectoralis major
pars abdominis

Humerus**

Rectus abdominis

Latissimus dorsi

Serratus anterior

Tendinous inscription

Obliquus externus

Iliac crest

Umbilicus

LATERAL VIEW

DEEP MUSCLES

LAYER II

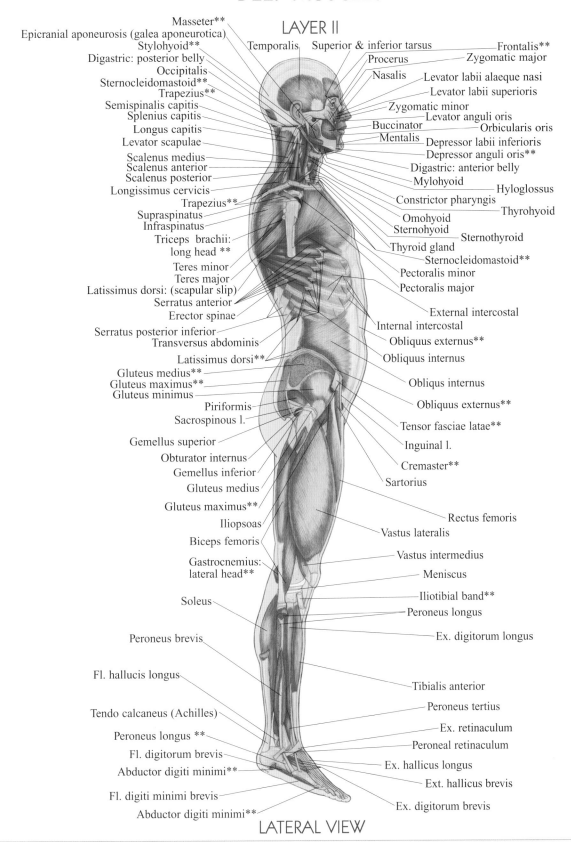

Masseter**
Epicranial aponeurosis (galea aponeurotica)
Stylohyoid**
Digastric: posterior belly
Occipitalis
Sternocleidomastoid**
Trapezius**
Semispinalis capitis
Splenius capitis
Longus capitis
Levator scapulae
Scalenus medius
Scalenus anterior
Scalenus posterior
Longissimus cervicis
Trapezius**
Supraspinatus
Infraspinatus
Triceps brachii: long head **
Teres minor
Teres major
Latissimus dorsi: (scapular slip)
Serratus anterior
Erector spinae
Serratus posterior inferior
Transversus abdominis
Latissimus dorsi**
Gluteus medius**
Gluteus maximus**
Gluteus minimus
Piriformis
Sacrospinous l.
Gemellus superior
Obturator internus
Gemellus inferior
Gluteus medius
Gluteus maximus**
Iliopsoas
Biceps femoris
Gastrocnemius: lateral head**
Soleus
Peroneus brevis
Fl. hallucis longus
Tendo calcaneus (Achilles)
Peroneus longus **
Fl. digitorum brevis
Abductor digiti minimi**
Fl. digiti minimi brevis
Abductor digiti minimi**

Temporalis
Superior & inferior tarsus
Procerus
Nasalis
Zygomatic minor
Buccinator
Mentalis

Frontalis**
Zygomatic major
Levator labii alaeque nasi
Levator labii superioris
Levator anguli oris
Orbicularis oris
Depressor labii inferioris
Depressor anguli oris**
Digastric: anterior belly
Mylohyoid
Hyloglossus
Constrictor pharyngis
Thyrohyoid
Omohyoid
Sternohyoid
Sternothyroid
Thyroid gland
Sternocleidomastoid**
Pectoralis minor
Pectoralis major
External intercostal
Internal intercostal
Obliquus externus**
Obliquus internus
Obliqus internus
Obliquus externus**
Tensor fasciae latae**
Inguinal l.
Cremaster**
Sartorius
Rectus femoris
Vastus lateralis
Vastus intermedius
Meniscus
Iliotibial band**
Peroneus longus
Ex. digitorum longus
Tibialis anterior
Peroneus tertius
Ex. retinaculum
Peroneal retinaculum
Ex. hallicus longus
Ext. hallicus brevis
Ex. digitorum brevis

LATERAL VIEW

DEEP MUSCLES

LAYER III

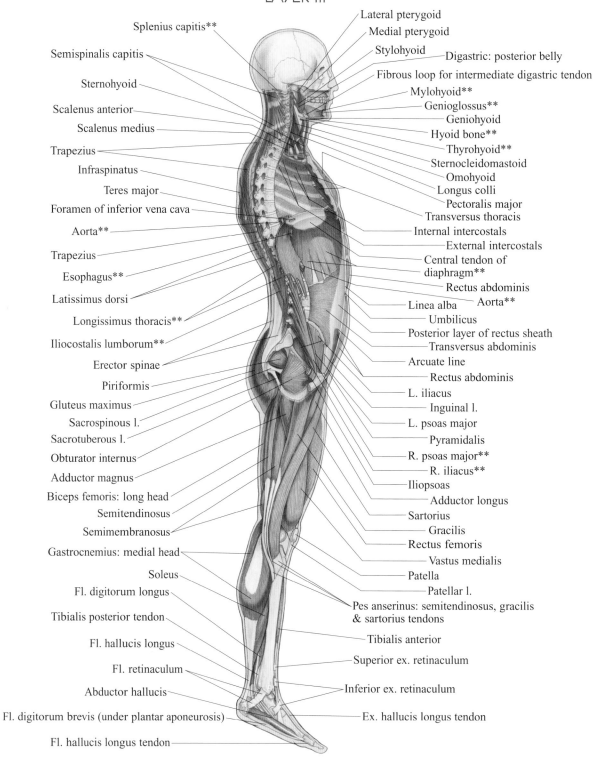

Splenius capitis**

Semispinalis capitis

Sternohyoid

Scalenus anterior

Scalenus medius

Trapezius

Infraspinatus

Teres major

Foramen of inferior vena cava

Aorta**

Trapezius

Esophagus**

Latissimus dorsi

Longissimus thoracis**

Iliocostalis lumborum**

Erector spinae

Piriformis

Gluteus maximus

Sacrospinous l.

Sacrotuberous l.

Obturator internus

Adductor magnus

Biceps femoris: long head

Semitendinosus

Semimembranosus

Gastrocnemius: medial head

Soleus

Fl. digitorum longus

Tibialis posterior tendon

Fl. hallucis longus

Fl. retinaculum

Abductor hallucis

Fl. digitorum brevis (under plantar aponeurosis)

Fl. hallucis longus tendon

Lateral pterygoid

Medial pterygoid

Stylohyoid

Digastric: posterior belly

Fibrous loop for intermediate digastric tendon

Mylohyoid**

Genioglossus**

Geniohyoid

Hyoid bone**

Thyrohyoid**

Sternocleidomastoid

Omohyoid

Longus colli

Pectoralis major

Transversus thoracis

Internal intercostals

External intercostals

Central tendon of diaphragm**

Rectus abdominis

Linea alba

Aorta**

Umbilicus

Posterior layer of rectus sheath

Transversus abdominis

Arcuate line

Rectus abdominis

L. iliacus

Inguinal l.

L. psoas major

Pyramidalis

R. psoas major**

R. iliacus**

Iliopsoas

Adductor longus

Sartorius

Gracilis

Rectus femoris

Vastus medialis

Patella

Patellar l.

Pes anserinus: semitendinosus, gracilis & sartorius tendons

Tibialis anterior

Superior ex. retinaculum

Inferior ex. retinaculum

Ex. hallucis longus tendon

LATERAL VIEW (MEDIAL LEG)

HEAD MUSCLES

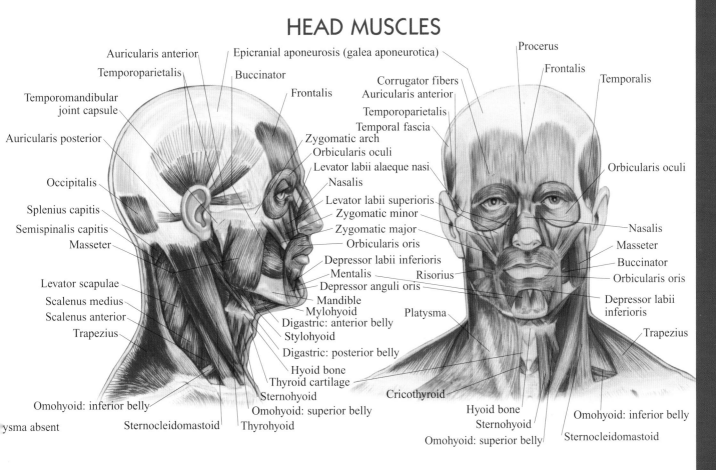

Auricularis anterior
Temporoparietalis
Temporomandibular joint capsule
Auricularis posterior
Occipitalis
Splenius capitis
Semispinalis capitis
Masseter
Levator scapulae
Scalenus medius
Scalenus anterior
Trapezius
Omohyoid: inferior belly
ysma absent
Sternocleidomastoid

Epicranial aponeurosis (galea aponeurotica)
Buccinator
Frontalis
Zygomatic arch
Orbicularis oculi
Levator labii alaeque nasi
Nasalis
Levator labii superioris
Zygomatic minor
Zygomatic major
Orbicularis oris
Depressor labii inferioris
Mentalis
Depressor anguli oris
Mandible
Mylohyoid
Digastric: anterior belly
Stylohyoid
Digastric: posterior belly
Hyoid bone
Thyroid cartilage
Sternohyoid
Omohyoid: superior belly
Thyrohyoid

Procerus
Frontalis
Temporalis
Corrugator fibers
Auricularis anterior
Temporoparietalis
Temporal fascia
Orbicularis oculi
Nasalis
Masseter
Buccinator
Orbicularis oris
Depressor labii inferioris
Trapezius
Omohyoid: inferior belly
Sternocleidomastoid

Risorius
Platysma
Cricothyroid
Hyoid bone
Sternohyoid
Omohyoid: superior belly

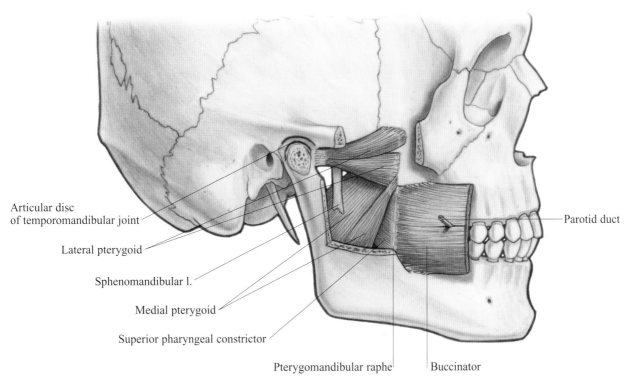

Articular disc of temporomandibular joint
Lateral pterygoid
Sphenomandibular l.
Medial pterygoid
Superior pharyngeal constrictor
Pterygomandibular raphe
Buccinator
Parotid duct

MUSCLES OF THE EYE

EXTRINSIC EYE MUSCLES

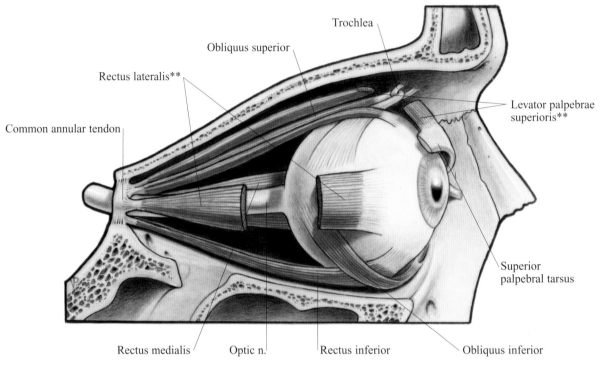

Trochlea

Obliquus superior

Rectus lateralis**

Common annular tendon

Levator palpebrae superioris**

Superior palpebral tarsus

Rectus medialis

Optic n.

Rectus inferior

Obliquus inferior

RIGHT LATERAL VIEW

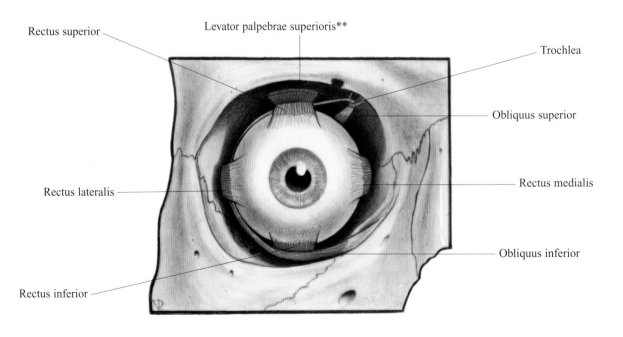

Rectus superior

Levator palpebrae superioris**

Trochlea

Obliquus superior

Rectus lateralis

Rectus medialis

Obliquus inferior

Rectus inferior

ANTERIOR VIEW

DEEP NECK MUSCLE

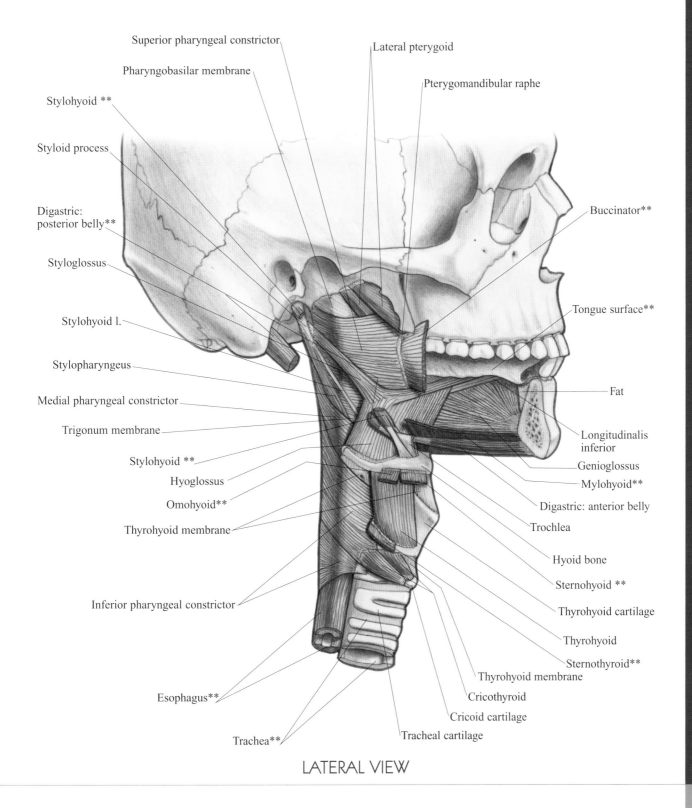

Superior pharyngeal constrictor

Pharyngobasilar membrane

Stylohyoid **

Styloid process

Digastric:
posterior belly**

Styloglossus

Stylohyoid l.

Stylopharyngeus

Medial pharyngeal constrictor

Trigonum membrane

Stylohyoid **

Hyoglossus

Omohyoid**

Thyrohyoid membrane

Inferior pharyngeal constrictor

Esophagus**

Trachea**

Lateral pterygoid

Pterygomandibular raphe

Buccinator**

Tongue surface**

Fat

Longitudinalis
inferior

Genioglossus

Mylohyoid**

Digastric: anterior belly

Trochlea

Hyoid bone

Sternohyoid **

Thyrohyoid cartilage

Thyrohyoid

Sternothyroid**

Thyrohyoid membrane

Cricothyroid

Cricoid cartilage

Tracheal cartilage

LATERAL VIEW

MUSCLES OF RESPIRATION

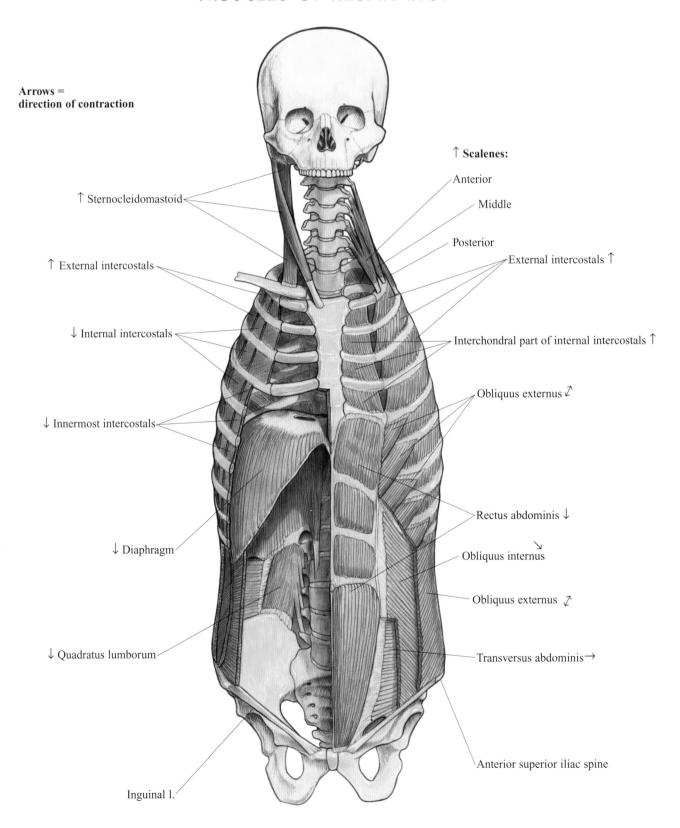

**Arrows =
direction of contraction**

↑ Sternocleidomastoid

↑ External intercostals

↓ Internal intercostals

↓ Innermost intercostals

↓ Diaphragm

↓ Quadratus lumborum

Inguinal l.

↑ **Scalenes:**

Anterior

Middle

Posterior

External intercostals ↑

Interchondral part of internal intercostals ↑

Obliquus externus ↙↗

Rectus abdominis ↓

Obliquus internus ↘

Obliquus externus ↙↗

Transversus abdominis →

Anterior superior iliac spine

COMPONENTS OF THE HAND
DORSAL VIEW

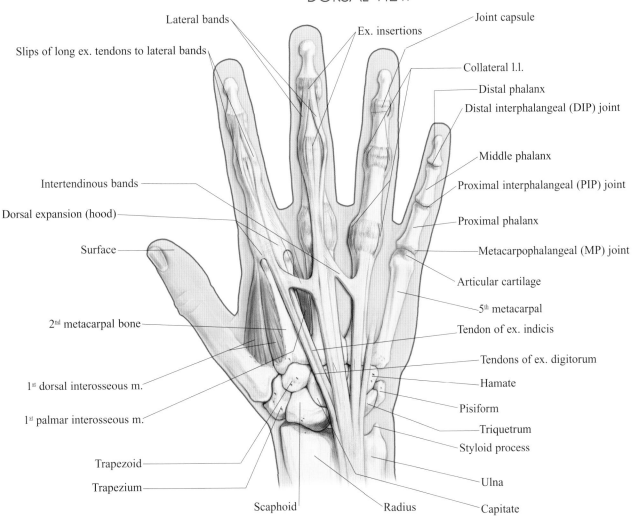

Lateral bands

Ex. insertions

Joint capsule

Slips of long ex. tendons to lateral bands

Collateral l.l.

Distal phalanx

Distal interphalangeal (DIP) joint

Middle phalanx

Proximal interphalangeal (PIP) joint

Intertendinous bands

Proximal phalanx

Dorsal expansion (hood)

Metacarpophalangeal (MP) joint

Surface

Articular cartilage

5th metacarpal

2nd metacarpal bone

Tendon of ex. indicis

Tendons of ex. digitorum

1st dorsal interosseous m.

Hamate

1st palmar interosseous m.

Pisiform

Triquetrum

Styloid process

Trapezoid

Trapezium

Ulna

Scaphoid

Radius

Capitate

COMPONENTS OF THE FINGER
CROSS SECTION

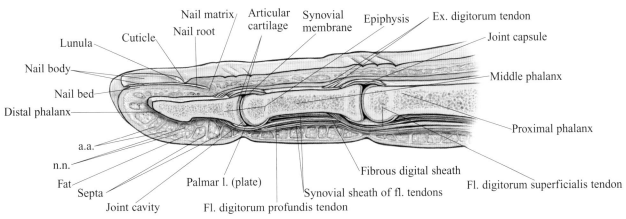

Nail matrix

Articular cartilage

Synovial membrane

Epiphysis

Ex. digitorum tendon

Nail root

Joint capsule

Lunula

Cuticle

Nail body

Middle phalanx

Nail bed

Distal phalanx

Proximal phalanx

a.a.

n.n.

Fat

Septa

Joint cavity

Palmar l. (plate)

Fl. digitorum profundis tendon

Synovial sheath of fl. tendons

Fibrous digital sheath

Fl. digitorum superficialis tendon

ARM & HAND MUSCLES

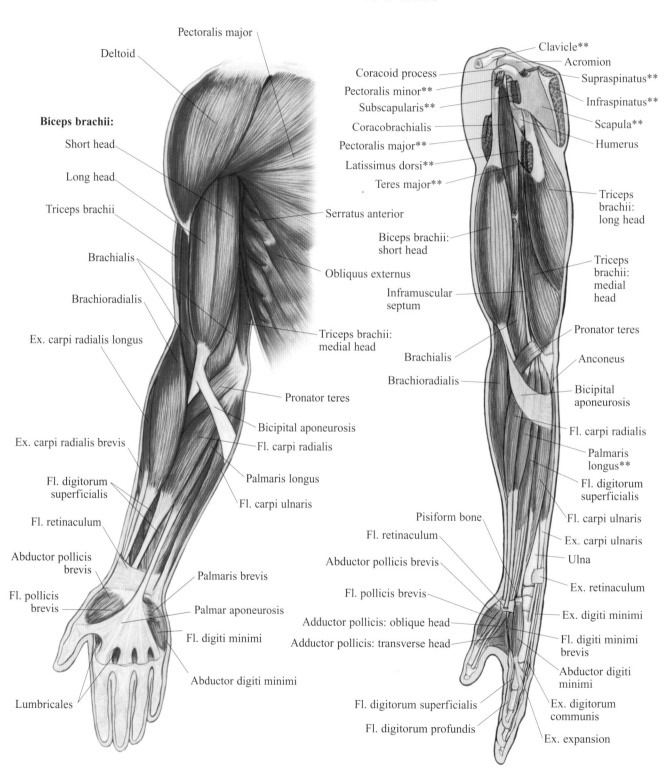

Pectoralis major

Deltoid

Biceps brachii:

Short head

Long head

Triceps brachii

Brachialis

Brachioradialis

Ex. carpi radialis longus

Ex. carpi radialis brevis

Fl. digitorum superficialis

Fl. retinaculum

Abductor pollicis brevis

Fl. pollicis brevis

Lumbricales

Serratus anterior

Obliquus externus

Triceps brachii: medial head

Pronator teres

Bicipital aponeurosis

Fl. carpi radialis

Palmaris longus

Fl. carpi ulnaris

Palmaris brevis

Palmar aponeurosis

Fl. digiti minimi

Abductor digiti minimi

Clavicle**

Acromion

Coracoid process

Pectoralis minor**

Subscapularis**

Coracobrachialis

Pectoralis major**

Latissimus dorsi**

Teres major**

Supraspinatus**

Infraspinatus**

Scapula**

Humerus

Triceps brachii: long head

Biceps brachii: short head

Inframuscular septum

Brachialis

Brachioradialis

Triceps brachii: medial head

Pronator teres

Anconeus

Bicipital aponeurosis

Fl. carpi radialis

Palmaris longus**

Fl. digitorum superficialis

Fl. carpi ulnaris

Ex. carpi ulnaris

Ulna

Ex. retinaculum

Ex. digiti minimi

Fl. digiti minimi brevis

Abductor digiti minimi

Ex. digitorum communis

Ex. expansion

Pisiform bone

Fl. retinaculum

Abductor pollicis brevis

Fl. pollicis brevis

Adductor pollicis: oblique head

Adductor pollicis: transverse head

Fl. digitorum superficialis

Fl. digitorum profundis

ANTERIOR VIEW

MEDIAL VIEW

ARM & HAND MUSCLES

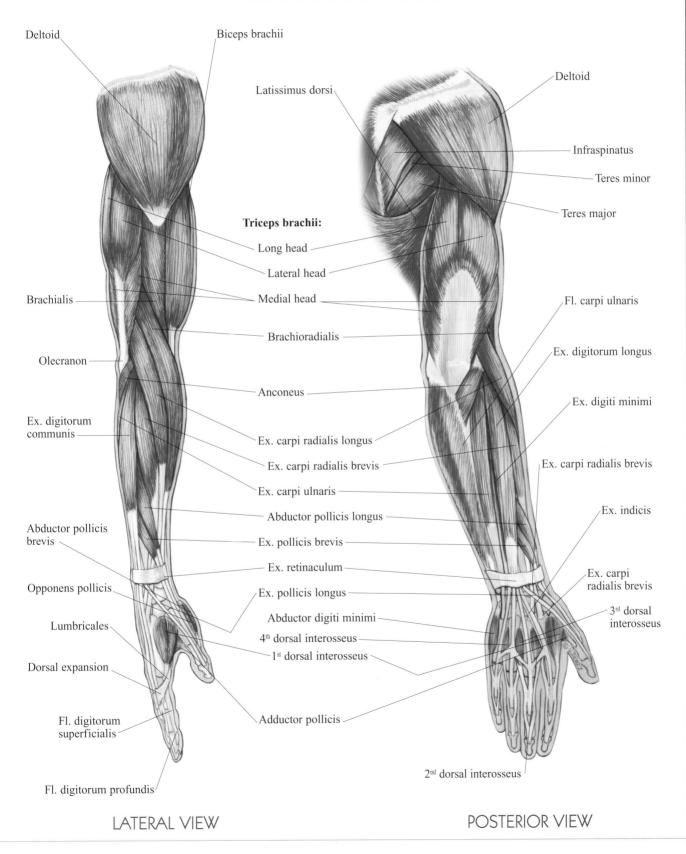

Deltoid

Biceps brachii

Latissimus dorsi

Deltoid

Infraspinatus

Teres minor

Teres major

Triceps brachii:

Long head

Lateral head

Brachialis

Medial head

Brachioradialis

Fl. carpi ulnaris

Olecranon

Ex. digitorum longus

Anconeus

Ex. digiti minimi

Ex. digitorum
communis

Ex. carpi radialis longus

Ex. carpi radialis brevis

Ex. carpi radialis brevis

Ex. carpi ulnaris

Abductor pollicis longus

Ex. indicis

Abductor pollicis
brevis

Ex. pollicis brevis

Ex. retinaculum

Ex. carpi
radialis brevis

Opponens pollicis

Ex. pollicis longus

3rd dorsal
interosseus

Lumbricales

Abductor digiti minimi

4th dorsal interosseus

Dorsal expansion

1st dorsal interosseus

Fl. digitorum
superficialis

Adductor pollicis

Fl. digitorum profundis

2nd dorsal interosseus

LATERAL VIEW

POSTERIOR VIEW

77

PALMAR HAND

LAYER I

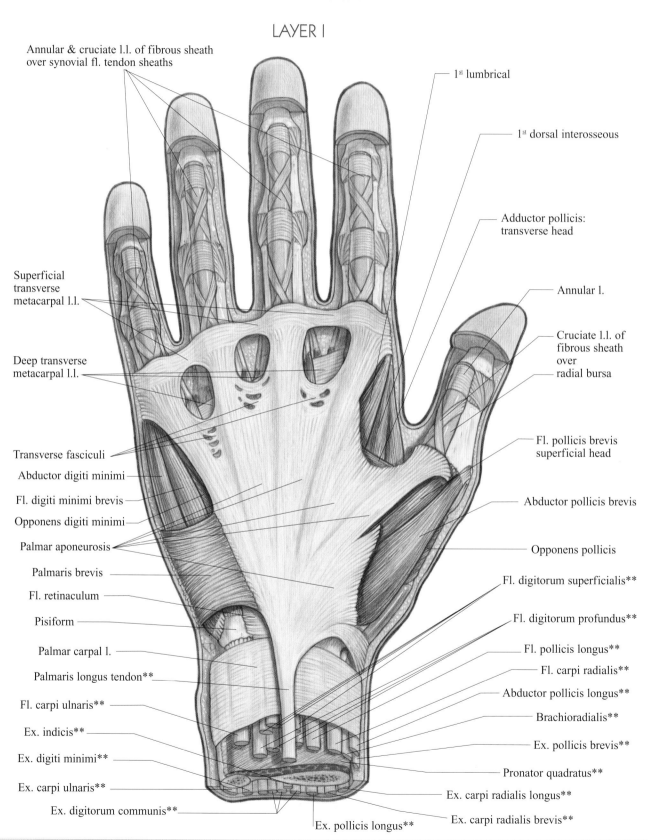

Annular & cruciate l.l. of fibrous sheath over synovial fl. tendon sheaths

1st lumbrical

1st dorsal interosseous

Adductor pollicis: transverse head

Superficial transverse metacarpal l.l.

Annular l.

Cruciate l.l. of fibrous sheath over radial bursa

Deep transverse metacarpal l.l.

Fl. pollicis brevis superficial head

Transverse fasciculi

Abductor digiti minimi

Fl. digiti minimi brevis

Opponens digiti minimi

Abductor pollicis brevis

Opponens pollicis

Palmar aponeurosis

Palmaris brevis

Fl. retinaculum

Fl. digitorum superficialis**

Pisiform

Fl. digitorum profundus**

Palmar carpal l.

Fl. pollicis longus**

Palmaris longus tendon**

Fl. carpi radialis**

Abductor pollicis longus**

Fl. carpi ulnaris**

Brachioradialis**

Ex. indicis**

Ex. pollicis brevis**

Ex. digiti minimi**

Pronator quadratus**

Ex. carpi ulnaris**

Ex. carpi radialis longus**

Ex. digitorum communis**

Ex. carpi radialis brevis**

Ex. pollicis longus**

PALMAR HAND

LAYER II

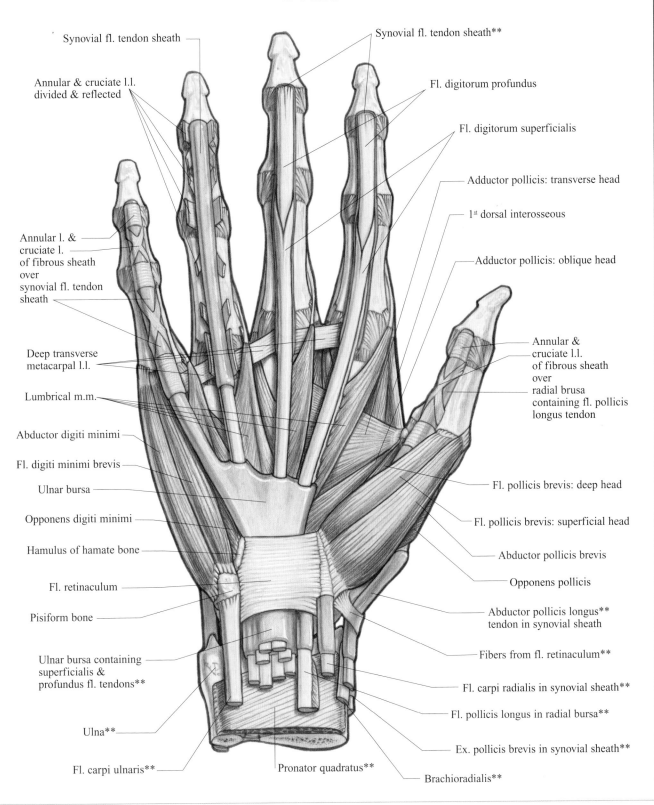

Synovial fl. tendon sheath

Synovial fl. tendon sheath**

Annular & cruciate l.l.
divided & reflected

Fl. digitorum profundus

Fl. digitorum superficialis

Adductor pollicis: transverse head

1ˢᵗ dorsal interosseous

Adductor pollicis: oblique head

Annular l. &
cruciate l.
of fibrous sheath
over
synovial fl. tendon
sheath

Annular &
cruciate l.l.
of fibrous sheath
over
radial brusa
containing fl. pollicis
longus tendon

Deep transverse
metacarpal l.l.

Lumbrical m.m.

Abductor digiti minimi

Fl. digiti minimi brevis

Ulnar bursa

Opponens digiti minimi

Hamulus of hamate bone

Fl. retinaculum

Pisiform bone

Ulnar bursa containing
superficialis &
profundus fl. tendons**

Ulna**

Fl. carpi ulnaris**

Pronator quadratus**

Fl. pollicis brevis: deep head

Fl. pollicis brevis: superficial head

Abductor pollicis brevis

Opponens pollicis

Abductor pollicis longus**
tendon in synovial sheath

Fibers from fl. retinaculum**

Fl. carpi radialis in synovial sheath**

Fl. pollicis longus in radial bursa**

Ex. pollicis brevis in synovial sheath**

Brachioradialis**

PALMAR HAND
LAYER III

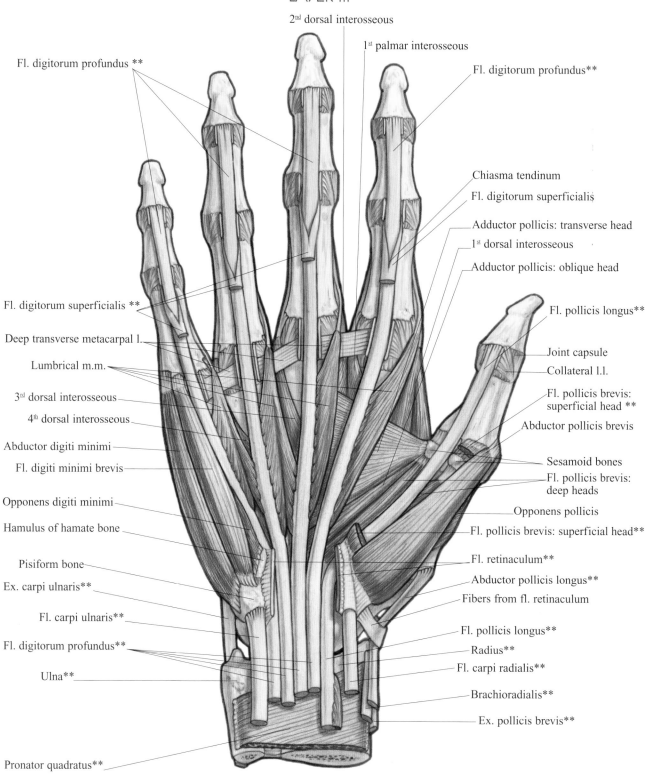

2nd dorsal interosseous

1st palmar interosseous

Fl. digitorum profundus **

Fl. digitorum profundus**

Chiasma tendinum

Fl. digitorum superficialis

Adductor pollicis: transverse head

1st dorsal interosseous

Adductor pollicis: oblique head

Fl. pollicis longus**

Joint capsule

Collateral l.l.

Fl. pollicis brevis: superficial head **

Abductor pollicis brevis

Sesamoid bones

Fl. pollicis brevis: deep heads

Opponens pollicis

Fl. pollicis brevis: superficial head**

Fl. retinaculum**

Abductor pollicis longus**

Fibers from fl. retinaculum

Fl. pollicis longus**

Radius**

Fl. carpi radialis**

Brachioradialis**

Ex. pollicis brevis**

Fl. digitorum superficialis **

Deep transverse metacarpal l.

Lumbrical m.m.

3rd dorsal interosseous

4th dorsal interosseous

Abductor digiti minimi

Fl. digiti minimi brevis

Opponens digiti minimi

Hamulus of hamate bone

Pisiform bone

Ex. carpi ulnaris**

Fl. carpi ulnaris**

Fl. digitorum profundus**

Ulna**

Pronator quadratus**

PALMAR HAND

LAYER IV

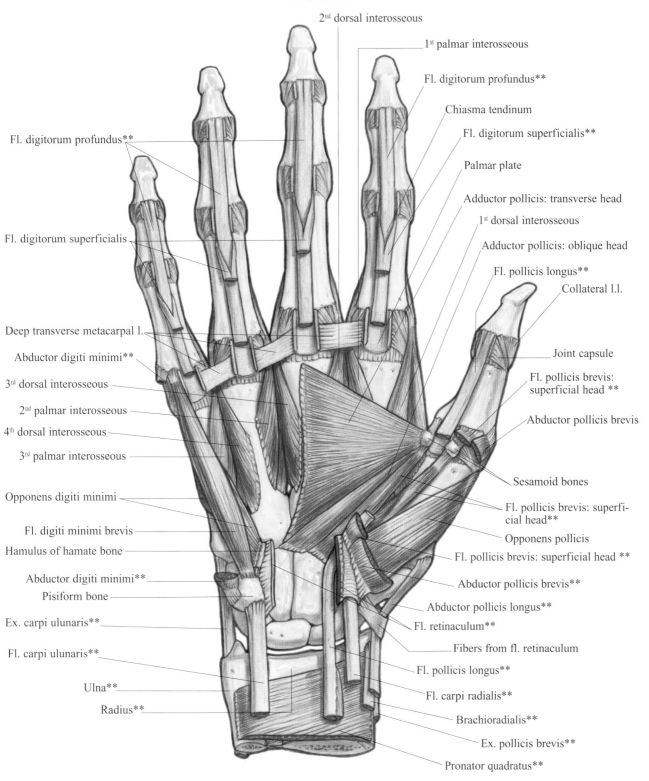

2nd dorsal interosseous

1st palmar interosseous

Fl. digitorum profundus**

Chiasma tendinum

Fl. digitorum superficialis**

Palmar plate

Adductor pollicis: transverse head

1st dorsal interosseous

Adductor pollicis: oblique head

Fl. pollicis longus**

Collateral l.l.

Joint capsule

Fl. pollicis brevis: superficial head **

Abductor pollicis brevis

Sesamoid bones

Fl. pollicis brevis: superficial head**

Opponens pollicis

Fl. pollicis brevis: superficial head **

Abductor pollicis brevis**

Abductor pollicis longus**

Fl. retinaculum**

Fibers from fl. retinaculum

Fl. pollicis longus**

Fl. carpi radialis**

Brachioradialis**

Ex. pollicis brevis**

Pronator quadratus**

Fl. digitorum profundus**

Fl. digitorum superficialis

Deep transverse metacarpal l.

Abductor digiti minimi**

3rd dorsal interosseous

2nd palmar interosseous

4th dorsal interosseous

3rd palmar interosseous

Opponens digiti minimi

Fl. digiti minimi brevis

Hamulus of hamate bone

Abductor digiti minimi**

Pisiform bone

Ex. carpi ulunaris**

Fl. carpi ulunaris**

Ulna**

Radius**

PALMAR HAND

LAYER V

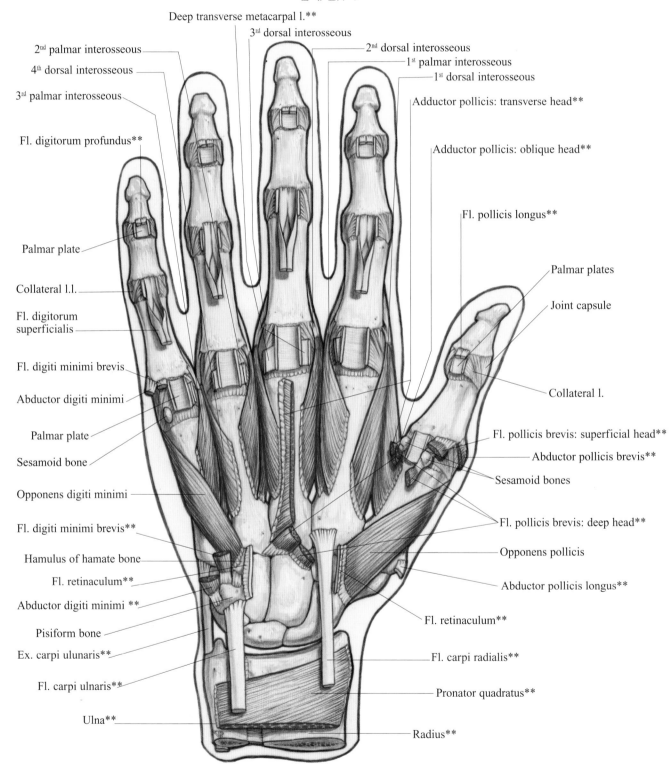

Deep transverse metacarpal l.**

3rd dorsal interosseous

2nd palmar interosseous

4th dorsal interosseous

3rd palmar interosseous

Fl. digitorum profundus**

Palmar plate

Collateral l.l.

Fl. digitorum superficialis

Fl. digiti minimi brevis

Abductor digiti minimi

Palmar plate

Sesamoid bone

Opponens digiti minimi

Fl. digiti minimi brevis**

Hamulus of hamate bone

Fl. retinaculum**

Abductor digiti minimi **

Pisiform bone

Ex. carpi ulunaris**

Fl. carpi ulnaris**

Ulna**

2nd dorsal interosseous

1st palmar interosseous

1st dorsal interosseous

Adductor pollicis: transverse head**

Adductor pollicis: oblique head**

Fl. pollicis longus**

Palmar plates

Joint capsule

Collateral l.

Fl. pollicis brevis: superficial head**

Abductor pollicis brevis**

Sesamoid bones

Fl. pollicis brevis: deep head**

Opponens pollicis

Abductor pollicis longus**

Fl. retinaculum**

Fl. carpi radialis**

Pronator quadratus**

Radius**

DORSAL HAND

LAYER I

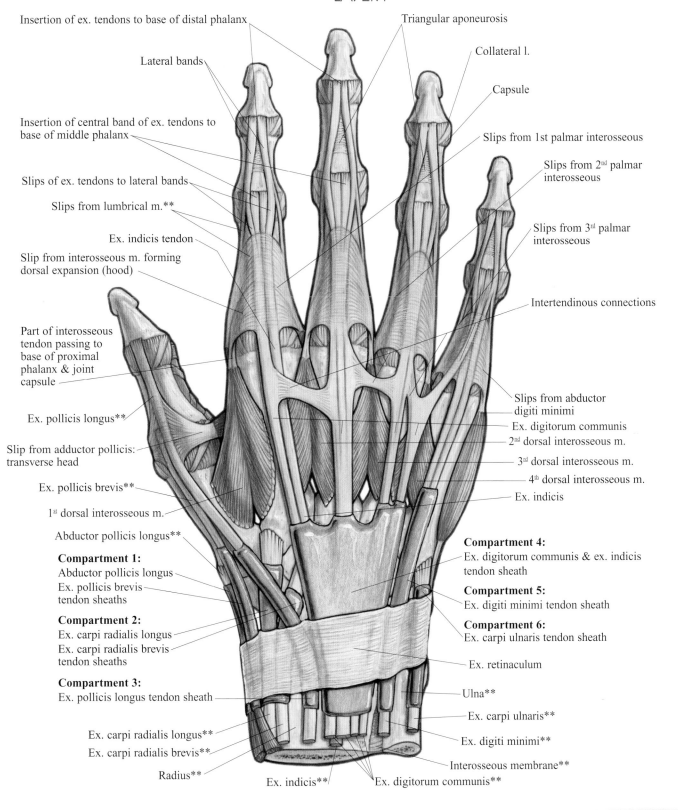

Insertion of ex. tendons to base of distal phalanx

Lateral bands

Insertion of central band of ex. tendons to base of middle phalanx

Slips of ex. tendons to lateral bands

Slips from lumbrical m.**

Ex. indicis tendon

Slip from interosseous m. forming dorsal expansion (hood)

Part of interosseous tendon passing to base of proximal phalanx & joint capsule

Ex. pollicis longus**

Slip from adductor pollicis: transverse head

Ex. pollicis brevis**

1st dorsal interosseous m.

Abductor pollicis longus**

Compartment 1:
Abductor pollicis longus
Ex. pollicis brevis
tendon sheaths

Compartment 2:
Ex. carpi radialis longus
Ex. carpi radialis brevis
tendon sheaths

Compartment 3:
Ex. pollicis longus tendon sheath

Ex. carpi radialis longus**

Ex. carpi radialis brevis**

Radius**

Ex. indicis**

Triangular aponeurosis

Collateral l.

Capsule

Slips from 1st palmar interosseous

Slips from 2nd palmar interosseous

Slips from 3rd palmar interosseous

Intertendinous connections

Slips from abductor digiti minimi

Ex. digitorum communis

2nd dorsal interosseous m.

3rd dorsal interosseous m.

4th dorsal interosseous m.

Ex. indicis

Compartment 4:
Ex. digitorum communis & ex. indicis tendon sheath

Compartment 5:
Ex. digiti minimi tendon sheath

Compartment 6:
Ex. carpi ulnaris tendon sheath

Ex. retinaculum

Ulna**

Ex. carpi ulnaris**

Ex. digiti minimi**

Interosseous membrane**

Ex. digitorum communis**

DORSAL HAND
LAYER II

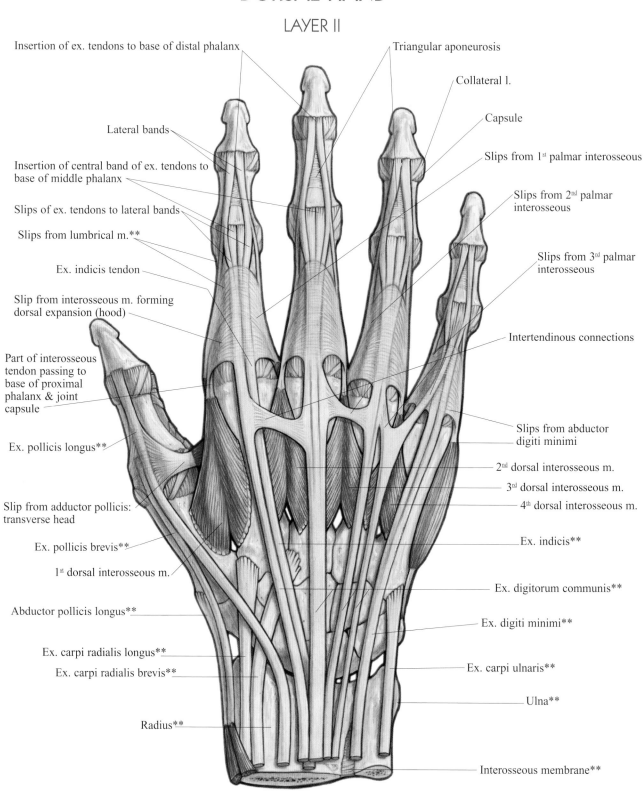

Insertion of ex. tendons to base of distal phalanx

Triangular aponeurosis

Collateral l.

Lateral bands

Capsule

Insertion of central band of ex. tendons to base of middle phalanx

Slips from 1st palmar interosseous

Slips of ex. tendons to lateral bands

Slips from 2nd palmar interosseous

Slips from lumbrical m.**

Slips from 3rd palmar interosseous

Ex. indicis tendon

Slip from interosseous m. forming dorsal expansion (hood)

Intertendinous connections

Part of interosseous tendon passing to base of proximal phalanx & joint capsule

Slips from abductor digiti minimi

Ex. pollicis longus**

2nd dorsal interosseous m.

3rd dorsal interosseous m.

4th dorsal interosseous m.

Slip from adductor pollicis: transverse head

Ex. indicis**

Ex. pollicis brevis**

Ex. digitorum communis**

1st dorsal interosseous m.

Abductor pollicis longus**

Ex. digiti minimi**

Ex. carpi radialis longus**

Ex. carpi ulnaris**

Ex. carpi radialis brevis**

Ulna**

Radius**

Interosseous membrane**

DORSAL HAND
LAYER III

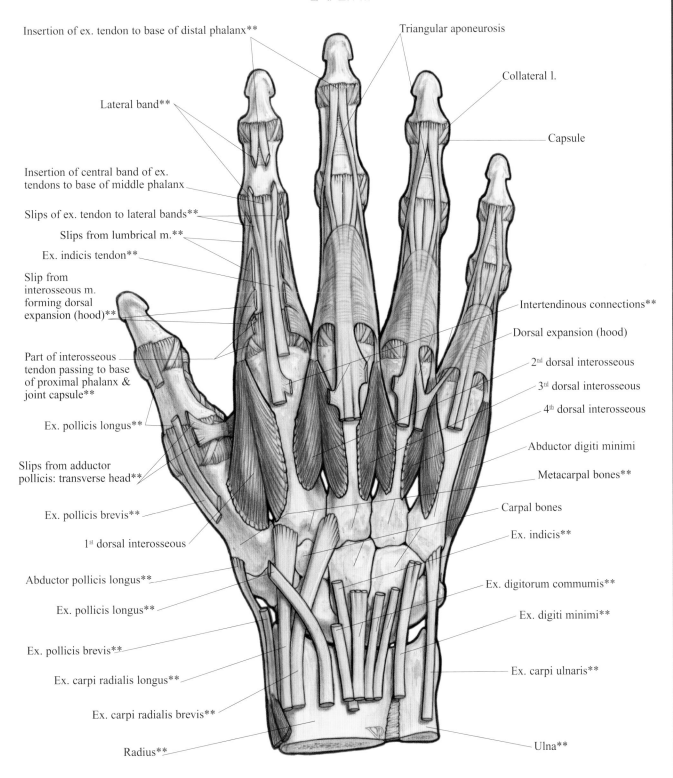

Insertion of ex. tendon to base of distal phalanx**

Triangular aponeurosis

Collateral l.

Lateral band**

Capsule

Insertion of central band of ex. tendons to base of middle phalanx

Slips of ex. tendon to lateral bands**

Slips from lumbrical m.**

Ex. indicis tendon**

Slip from interosseous m. forming dorsal expansion (hood)**

Intertendinous connections**

Dorsal expansion (hood)

2nd dorsal interosseous

3rd dorsal interosseous

4th dorsal interosseous

Part of interosseous tendon passing to base of proximal phalanx & joint capsule**

Abductor digiti minimi

Ex. pollicis longus**

Metacarpal bones**

Slips from adductor pollicis: transverse head**

Carpal bones

Ex. indicis**

Ex. pollicis brevis**

1st dorsal interosseous

Ex. digitorum commumis**

Abductor pollicis longus**

Ex. pollicis longus**

Ex. digiti minimi**

Ex. pollicis brevis**

Ex. carpi ulnaris**

Ex. carpi radialis longus**

Ex. carpi radialis brevis**

Radius**

Ulna**

MEDIAL HAND

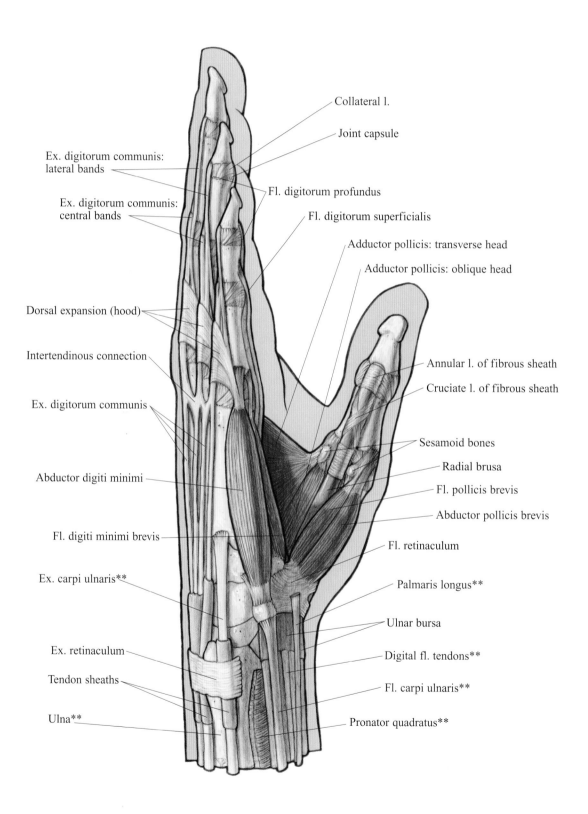

Collateral l.

Joint capsule

Ex. digitorum communis: lateral bands

Fl. digitorum profundus

Ex. digitorum communis: central bands

Fl. digitorum superficialis

Adductor pollicis: transverse head

Adductor pollicis: oblique head

Dorsal expansion (hood)

Intertendinous connection

Annular l. of fibrous sheath

Cruciate l. of fibrous sheath

Ex. digitorum communis

Sesamoid bones

Radial brusa

Abductor digiti minimi

Fl. pollicis brevis

Abductor pollicis brevis

Fl. digiti minimi brevis

Fl. retinaculum

Ex. carpi ulnaris**

Palmaris longus**

Ulnar bursa

Ex. retinaculum

Digital fl. tendons**

Tendon sheaths

Fl. carpi ulnaris**

Ulna**

Pronator quadratus**

LATERAL HAND

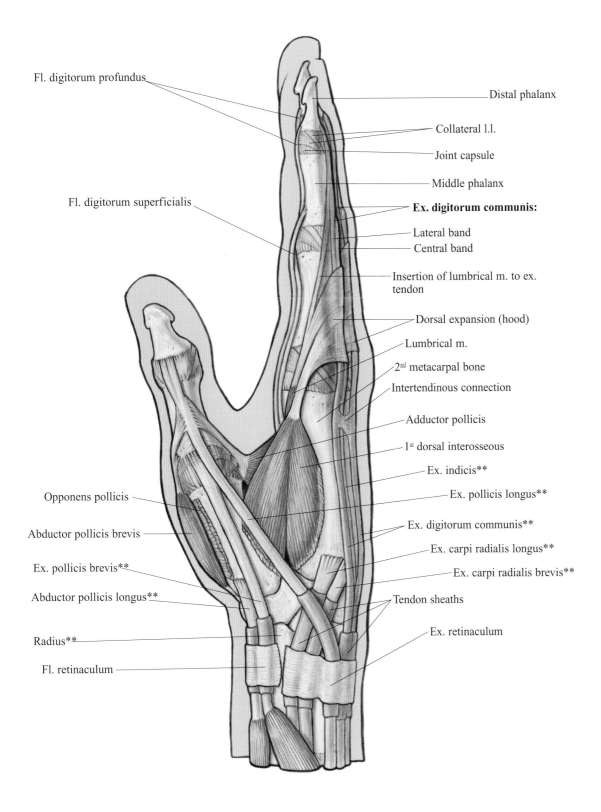

Fl. digitorum profundus

Distal phalanx

Collateral l.l.

Joint capsule

Middle phalanx

Fl. digitorum superficialis

Ex. digitorum communis:

Lateral band

Central band

Insertion of lumbrical m. to ex. tendon

Dorsal expansion (hood)

Lumbrical m.

2nd metacarpal bone

Intertendinous connection

Adductor pollicis

1st dorsal interosseous

Ex. indicis**

Ex. pollicis longus**

Opponens pollicis

Ex. digitorum communis**

Abductor pollicis brevis

Ex. carpi radialis longus**

Ex. pollicis brevis**

Ex. carpi radialis brevis**

Abductor pollicis longus**

Tendon sheaths

Radius**

Ex. retinaculum

Fl. retinaculum

LEG & FOOT SURFACE MUSCLES

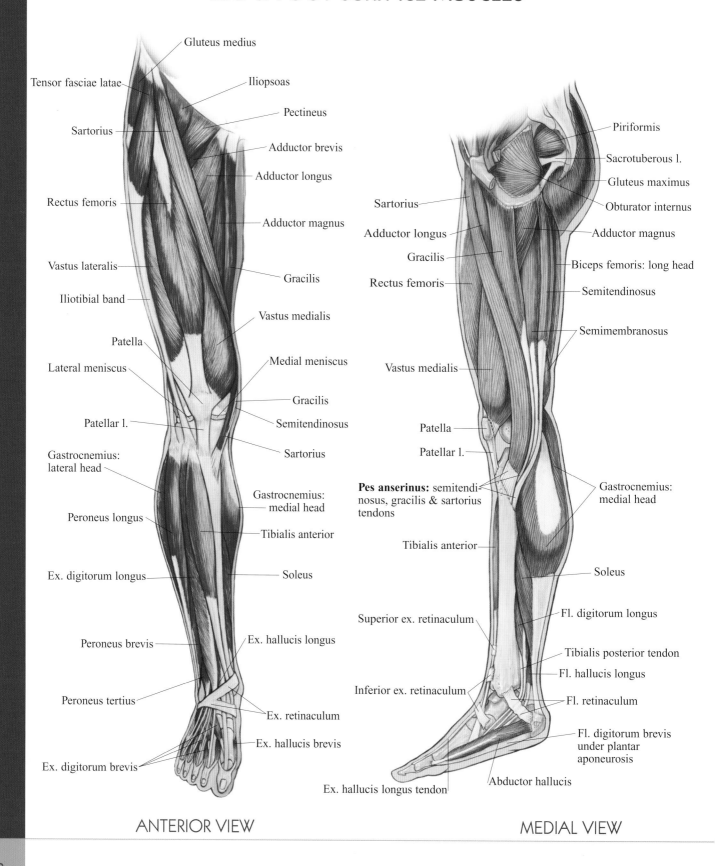

Gluteus medius

Tensor fasciae latae

Iliopsoas

Sartorius

Pectineus

Adductor brevis

Adductor longus

Rectus femoris

Adductor magnus

Vastus lateralis

Gracilis

Iliotibial band

Vastus medialis

Patella

Lateral meniscus

Medial meniscus

Patellar l.

Gracilis

Semitendinosus

Sartorius

Gastrocnemius: lateral head

Gastrocnemius: medial head

Peroneus longus

Tibialis anterior

Ex. digitorum longus

Soleus

Peroneus brevis

Ex. hallucis longus

Peroneus tertius

Ex. retinaculum

Ex. hallucis brevis

Ex. digitorum brevis

Piriformis

Sacrotuberous l.

Gluteus maximus

Obturator internus

Sartorius

Adductor magnus

Adductor longus

Biceps femoris: long head

Gracilis

Semitendinosus

Rectus femoris

Semimembranosus

Vastus medialis

Patella

Patellar l.

Gastrocnemius: medial head

Pes anserinus: semitendinosus, gracilis & sartorius tendons

Tibialis anterior

Soleus

Superior ex. retinaculum

Fl. digitorum longus

Tibialis posterior tendon

Fl. hallucis longus

Inferior ex. retinaculum

Fl. retinaculum

Fl. digitorum brevis under plantar aponeurosis

Ex. hallucis longus tendon

Abductor hallucis

ANTERIOR VIEW

MEDIAL VIEW

LEG & FOOT SURFACE MUSCLES

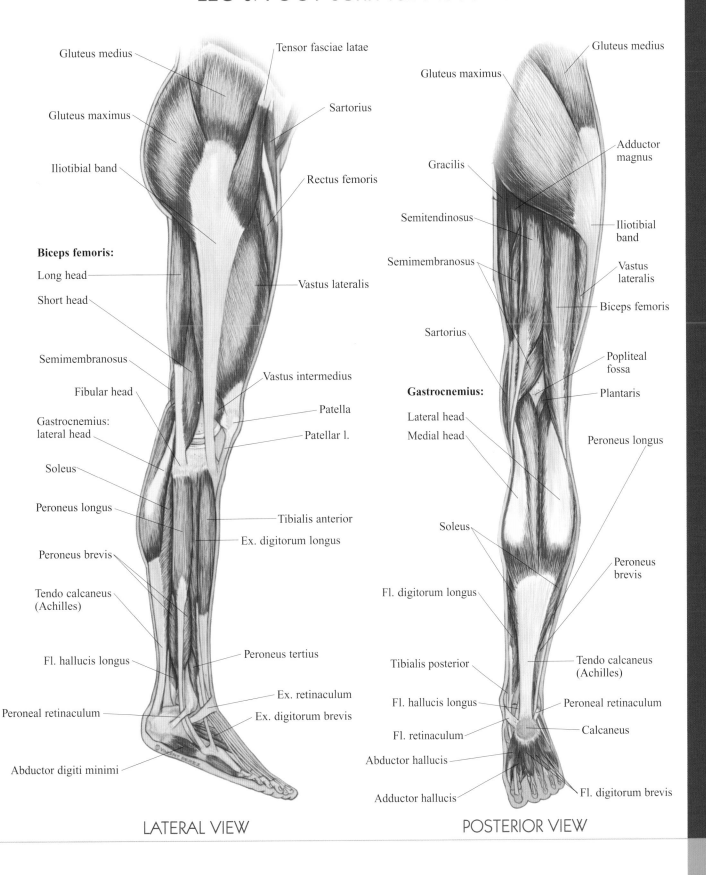

Gluteus medius

Tensor fasciae latae

Gluteus maximus

Sartorius

Iliotibial band

Rectus femoris

Biceps femoris:

Long head

Vastus lateralis

Short head

Semimembranosus

Fibular head

Vastus intermedius

Gastrocnemius:
lateral head

Patella

Soleus

Patellar l.

Peroneus longus

Peroneus brevis

Tibialis anterior

Tendo calcaneus
(Achilles)

Ex. digitorum longus

Fl. hallucis longus

Peroneus tertius

Peroneal retinaculum

Ex. retinaculum

Ex. digitorum brevis

Abductor digiti minimi

LATERAL VIEW

Gluteus medius

Gluteus maximus

Adductor
magnus

Gracilis

Iliotibial
band

Semitendinosus

Vastus
lateralis

Semimembranosus

Biceps femoris

Sartorius

Popliteal
fossa

Gastrocnemius:

Plantaris

Lateral head

Peroneus longus

Medial head

Soleus

Peroneus
brevis

Fl. digitorum longus

Tibialis posterior

Tendo calcaneus
(Achilles)

Fl. hallucis longus

Peroneal retinaculum

Fl. retinaculum

Calcaneus

Abductor hallucis

Adductor hallucis

Fl. digitorum brevis

POSTERIOR VIEW

DORSAL FOOT
LAYER I

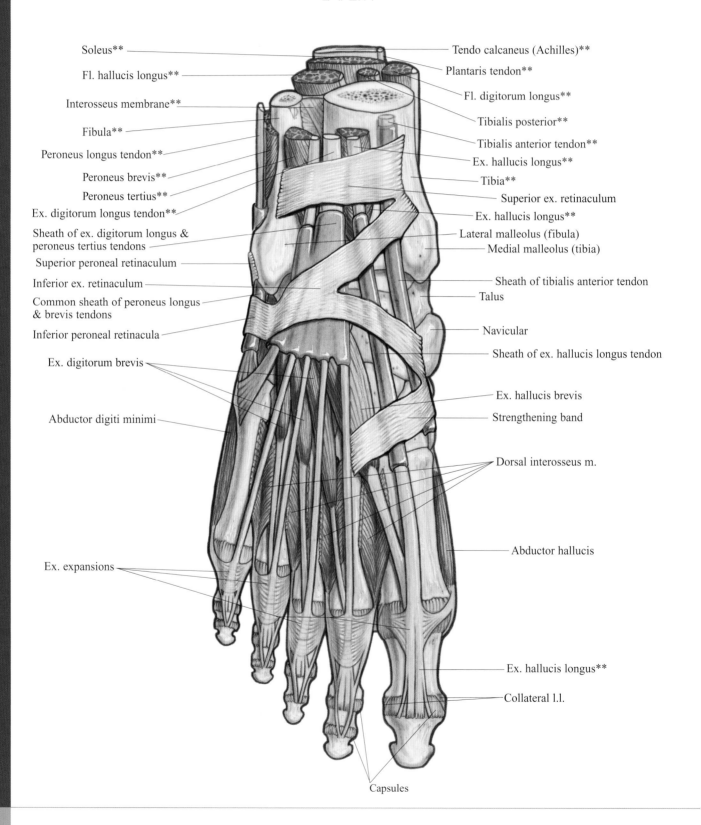

Soleus**

Fl. hallucis longus**

Interosseus membrane**

Fibula**

Peroneus longus tendon**

Peroneus brevis**

Peroneus tertius**

Ex. digitorum longus tendon**

Sheath of ex. digitorum longus &
peroneus tertius tendons

Superior peroneal retinaculum

Inferior ex. retinaculum

Common sheath of peroneus longus
& brevis tendons

Inferior peroneal retinacula

Ex. digitorum brevis

Abductor digiti minimi

Ex. expansions

Tendo calcaneus (Achilles)**

Plantaris tendon**

Fl. digitorum longus**

Tibialis posterior**

Tibialis anterior tendon**

Ex. hallucis longus**

Tibia**

Superior ex. retinaculum

Ex. hallucis longus**

Lateral malleolus (fibula)

Medial malleolus (tibia)

Sheath of tibialis anterior tendon

Talus

Navicular

Sheath of ex. hallucis longus tendon

Ex. hallucis brevis

Strengthening band

Dorsal interosseus m.

Abductor hallucis

Ex. hallucis longus**

Collateral l.l.

Capsules

DORSAL FOOT

LAYER II

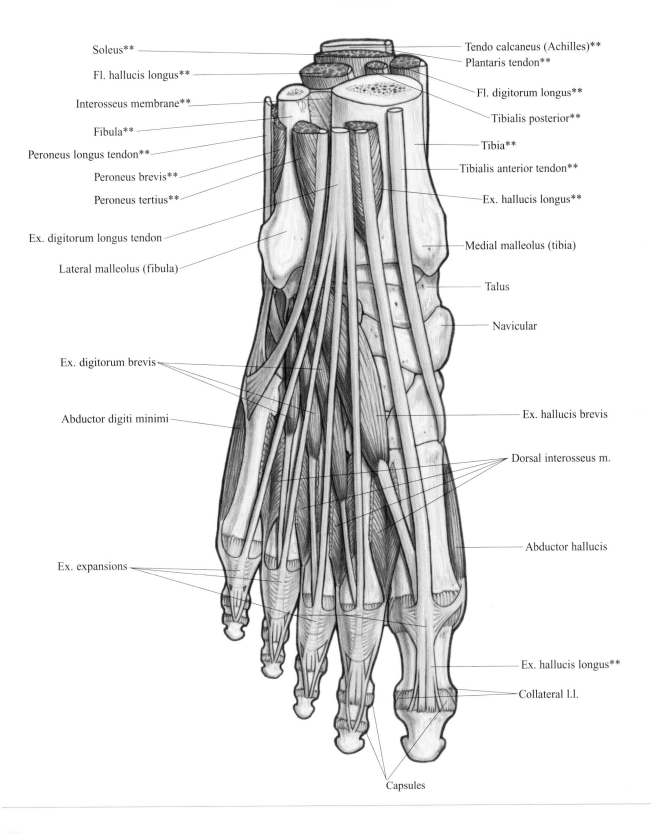

Soleus**

Fl. hallucis longus**

Interosseus membrane**

Fibula**

Peroneus longus tendon**

Peroneus brevis**

Peroneus tertius**

Ex. digitorum longus tendon

Lateral malleolus (fibula)

Ex. digitorum brevis

Abductor digiti minimi

Ex. expansions

Tendo calcaneus (Achilles)**

Plantaris tendon**

Fl. digitorum longus**

Tibialis posterior**

Tibia**

Tibialis anterior tendon**

Ex. hallucis longus**

Medial malleolus (tibia)

Talus

Navicular

Ex. hallucis brevis

Dorsal interosseus m.

Abductor hallucis

Ex. hallucis longus**

Collateral l.l.

Capsules

DORSAL FOOT

LAYER III

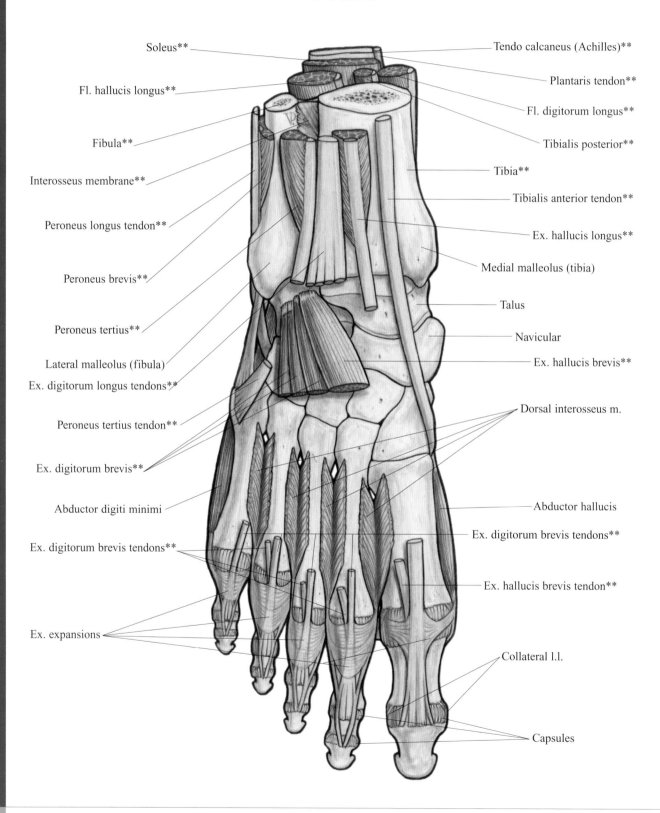

Soleus**

Fl. hallucis longus**

Fibula**

Interosseus membrane**

Peroneus longus tendon**

Peroneus brevis**

Peroneus tertius**

Lateral malleolus (fibula)

Ex. digitorum longus tendons**

Peroneus tertius tendon**

Ex. digitorum brevis**

Abductor digiti minimi

Ex. digitorum brevis tendons**

Ex. expansions

Tendo calcaneus (Achilles)**

Plantaris tendon**

Fl. digitorum longus**

Tibialis posterior**

Tibia**

Tibialis anterior tendon**

Ex. hallucis longus**

Medial malleolus (tibia)

Talus

Navicular

Ex. hallucis brevis**

Dorsal interosseus m.

Abductor hallucis

Ex. digitorum brevis tendons**

Ex. hallucis brevis tendon**

Collateral l.l.

Capsules

PLANTAR FOOT

LAYER I

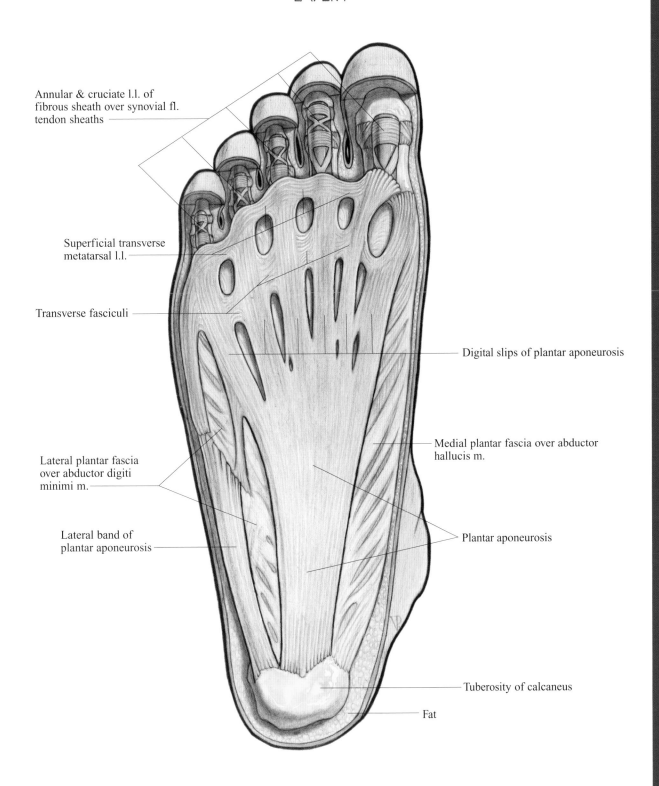

Annular & cruciate l.l. of fibrous sheath over synovial fl. tendon sheaths

Superficial transverse metatarsal l.l.

Transverse fasciculi

Digital slips of plantar aponeurosis

Medial plantar fascia over abductor hallucis m.

Lateral plantar fascia over abductor digiti minimi m.

Lateral band of plantar aponeurosis

Plantar aponeurosis

Tuberosity of calcaneus

Fat

PLANTAR FOOT

LAYER II

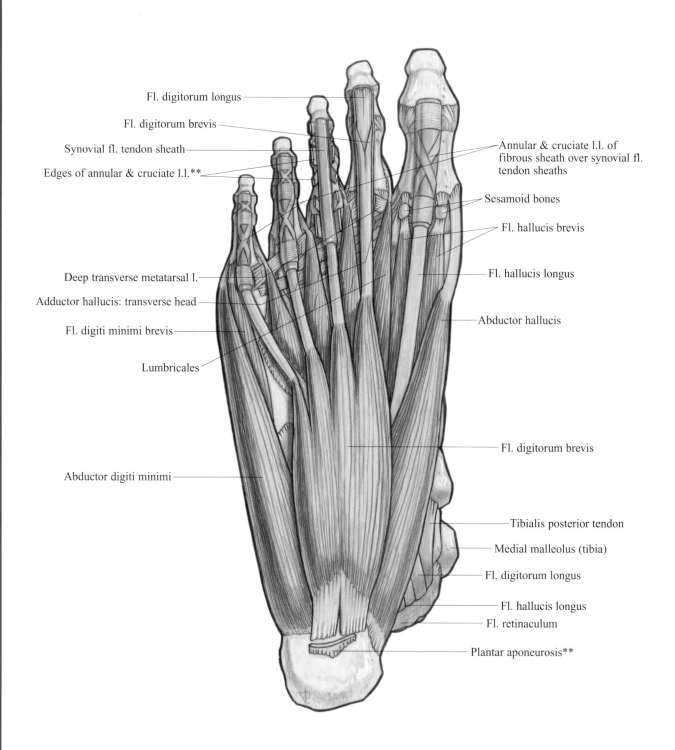

Fl. digitorum longus

Fl. digitorum brevis

Synovial fl. tendon sheath

Edges of annular & cruciate l.l.**

Deep transverse metatarsal l.

Adductor hallucis: transverse head

Fl. digiti minimi brevis

Lumbricales

Abductor digiti minimi

Annular & cruciate l.l. of fibrous sheath over synovial fl. tendon sheaths

Sesamoid bones

Fl. hallucis brevis

Fl. hallucis longus

Abductor hallucis

Fl. digitorum brevis

Tibialis posterior tendon

Medial malleolus (tibia)

Fl. digitorum longus

Fl. hallucis longus

Fl. retinaculum

Plantar aponeurosis**

PLANTAR FOOT

LAYER III

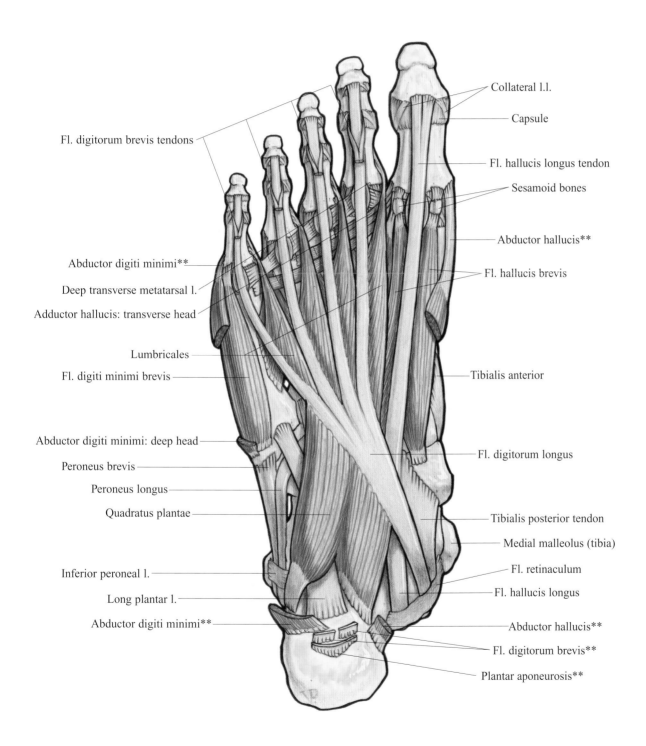

Fl. digitorum brevis tendons

Collateral l.l.

Capsule

Fl. hallucis longus tendon

Sesamoid bones

Abductor hallucis**

Abductor digiti minimi**

Deep transverse metatarsal l.

Adductor hallucis: transverse head

Fl. hallucis brevis

Lumbricales

Fl. digiti minimi brevis

Tibialis anterior

Abductor digiti minimi: deep head

Peroneus brevis

Peroneus longus

Quadratus plantae

Fl. digitorum longus

Tibialis posterior tendon

Medial malleolus (tibia)

Inferior peroneal l.

Long plantar l.

Abductor digiti minimi**

Fl. retinaculum

Fl. hallucis longus

Abductor hallucis**

Fl. digitorum brevis**

Plantar aponeurosis**

PLANTAR FOOT
LAYER IV

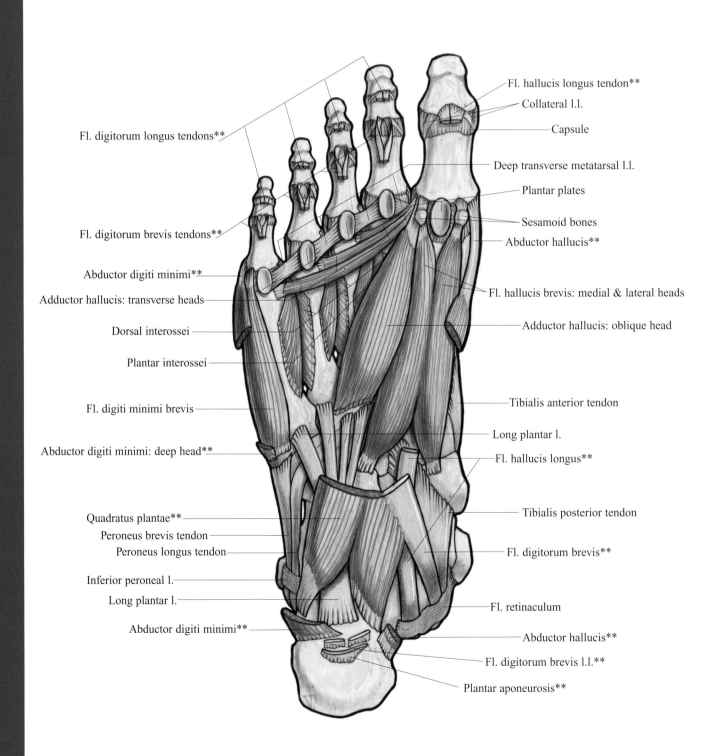

Fl. digitorum longus tendons**

Fl. hallucis longus tendon**

Collateral l.l.

Capsule

Deep transverse metatarsal l.l.

Plantar plates

Sesamoid bones

Abductor hallucis**

Fl. digitorum brevis tendons**

Abductor digiti minimi**

Adductor hallucis: transverse heads

Fl. hallucis brevis: medial & lateral heads

Dorsal interossei

Adductor hallucis: oblique head

Plantar interossei

Fl. digiti minimi brevis

Tibialis anterior tendon

Long plantar l.

Fl. hallucis longus**

Abductor digiti minimi: deep head**

Quadratus plantae**

Tibialis posterior tendon

Peroneus brevis tendon

Peroneus longus tendon

Fl. digitorum brevis**

Inferior peroneal l.

Long plantar l.

Fl. retinaculum

Abductor digiti minimi**

Abductor hallucis**

Fl. digitorum brevis l.l.**

Plantar aponeurosis**

PLANTAR FOOT

LAYER V

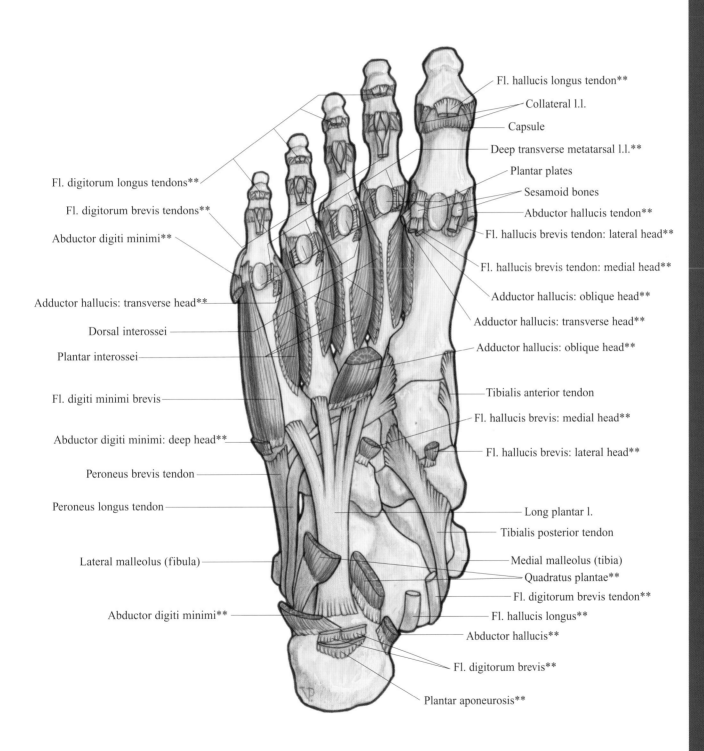

Fl. hallucis longus tendon**

Collateral l.l.

Capsule

Deep transverse metatarsal l.l.**

Plantar plates

Sesamoid bones

Abductor hallucis tendon**

Fl. hallucis brevis tendon: lateral head**

Fl. hallucis brevis tendon: medial head**

Adductor hallucis: oblique head**

Adductor hallucis: transverse head**

Adductor hallucis: oblique head**

Tibialis anterior tendon

Fl. hallucis brevis: medial head**

Fl. hallucis brevis: lateral head**

Long plantar l.

Tibialis posterior tendon

Medial malleolus (tibia)

Quadratus plantae**

Fl. digitorum brevis tendon**

Fl. hallucis longus**

Abductor hallucis**

Fl. digitorum brevis**

Plantar aponeurosis**

Fl. digitorum longus tendons**

Fl. digitorum brevis tendons**

Abductor digiti minimi**

Adductor hallucis: transverse head**

Dorsal interossei

Plantar interossei

Fl. digiti minimi brevis

Abductor digiti minimi: deep head**

Peroneus brevis tendon

Peroneus longus tendon

Lateral malleolus (fibula)

Abductor digiti minimi**

LATERAL FOOT

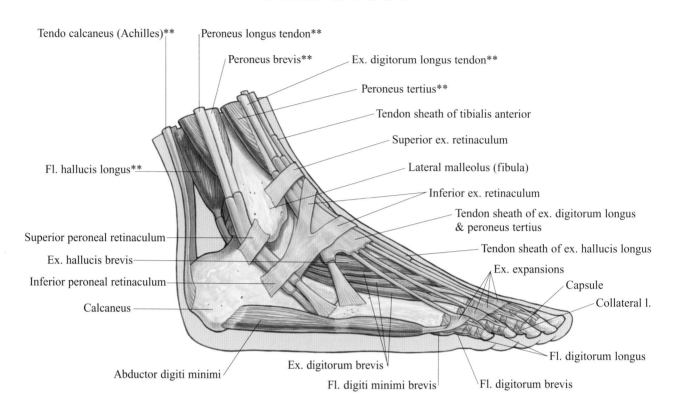

Tendo calcaneus (Achilles)**

Peroneus longus tendon**

Peroneus brevis**

Ex. digitorum longus tendon**

Peroneus tertius**

Tendon sheath of tibialis anterior

Superior ex. retinaculum

Lateral malleolus (fibula)

Fl. hallucis longus**

Inferior ex. retinaculum

Tendon sheath of ex. digitorum longus
& peroneus tertius

Tendon sheath of ex. hallucis longus

Superior peroneal retinaculum

Ex. hallucis brevis

Inferior peroneal retinaculum

Calcaneus

Ex. expansions

Capsule

Collateral l.

Fl. digitorum longus

Abductor digiti minimi

Ex. digitorum brevis

Fl. digiti minimi brevis

Fl. digitorum brevis

MEDIAL FOOT

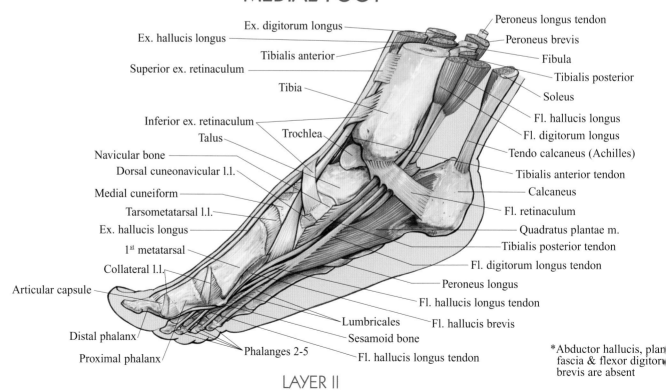

Ex. digitorum longus

Peroneus longus tendon

Ex. hallucis longus

Peroneus brevis

Tibialis anterior

Fibula

Superior ex. retinaculum

Tibialis posterior

Tibia

Soleus

Inferior ex. retinaculum

Fl. hallucis longus

Talus

Trochlea

Fl. digitorum longus

Navicular bone

Tendo calcaneus (Achilles)

Dorsal cuneonavicular l.l.

Tibialis anterior tendon

Medial cuneiform

Calcaneus

Tarsometatarsal l.l.

Fl. retinaculum

Ex. hallucis longus

Quadratus plantae m.

1st metatarsal

Tibialis posterior tendon

Collateral l.l.

Fl. digitorum longus tendon

Articular capsule

Peroneus longus

Fl. hallucis longus tendon

Lumbricales

Fl. hallucis brevis

Distal phalanx

Sesamoid bone

Proximal phalanx

Phalanges 2-5

Fl. hallucis longus tendon

*Abductor hallucis, plan
fascia & flexor digitor
brevis are absent

LAYER II

MUSCLE MICROSTRUCTURE
EXTENSOR INDICIS

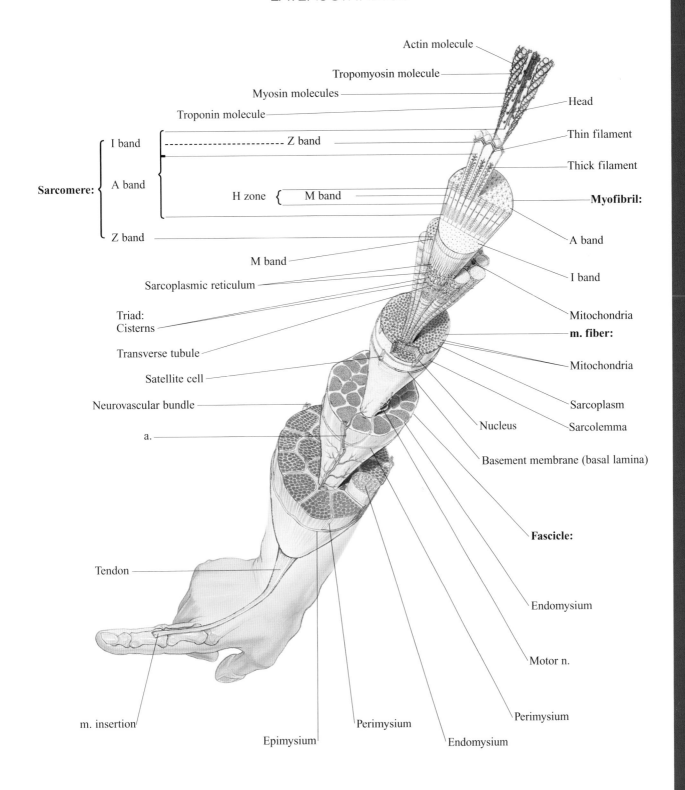

Actin molecule

Tropomyosin molecule

Myosin molecules

Troponin molecule

Head

I band

A band — Z band

Thin filament

Thick filament

Sarcomere:

H zone — M band

Myofibril:

Z band

A band

M band

I band

Sarcoplasmic reticulum

Mitochondria

Triad:
Cisterns

m. fiber:

Transverse tubule

Mitochondria

Satellite cell

Sarcoplasm

Neurovascular bundle

Nucleus

Sarcolemma

a.

Basement membrane (basal lamina)

Fascicle:

Tendon

Endomysium

Motor n.

m. insertion

Perimysium

Perimysium

Epimysium

Endomysium

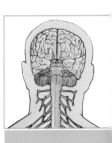

6

NERVOUS SYSTEM

NERVOUS SYSTEM

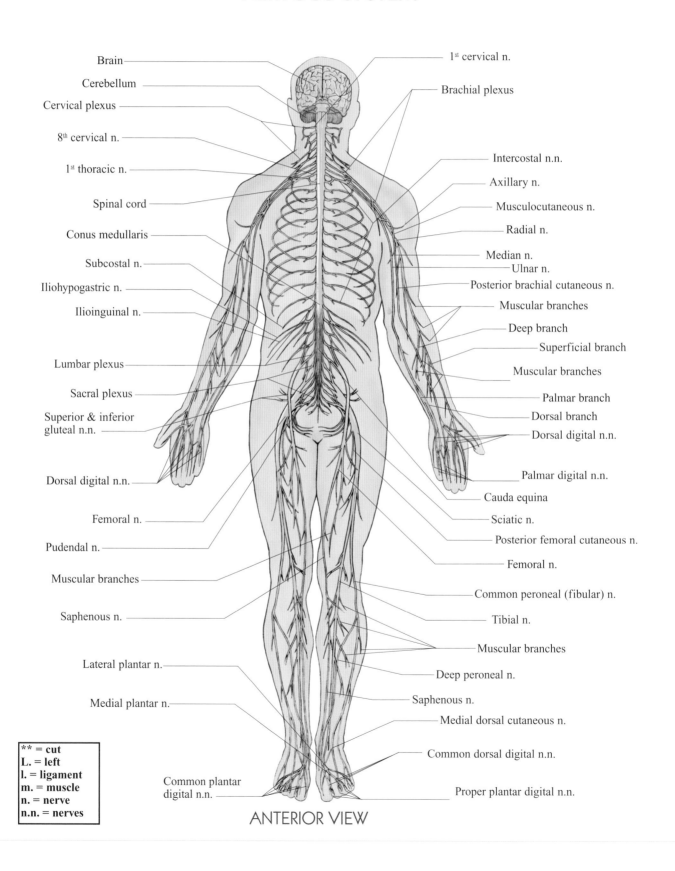

Brain

Cerebellum

Cervical plexus

8th cervical n.

1st thoracic n.

Spinal cord

Conus medullaris

Subcostal n.

Iliohypogastric n.

Ilioinguinal n.

Lumbar plexus

Sacral plexus

Superior & inferior gluteal n.n.

Dorsal digital n.n.

Femoral n.

Pudendal n.

Muscular branches

Saphenous n.

Lateral plantar n.

Medial plantar n.

Common plantar digital n.n.

1st cervical n.

Brachial plexus

Intercostal n.n.

Axillary n.

Musculocutaneous n.

Radial n.

Median n.

Ulnar n.

Posterior brachial cutaneous n.

Muscular branches

Deep branch

Superficial branch

Muscular branches

Palmar branch

Dorsal branch

Dorsal digital n.n.

Palmar digital n.n.

Cauda equina

Sciatic n.

Posterior femoral cutaneous n.

Femoral n.

Common peroneal (fibular) n.

Tibial n.

Muscular branches

Deep peroneal n.

Saphenous n.

Medial dorsal cutaneous n.

Common dorsal digital n.n.

Proper plantar digital n.n.

** = cut
L. = left
l. = ligament
m. = muscle
n. = nerve
n.n. = nerves

ANTERIOR VIEW

NERVOUS SYSTEM

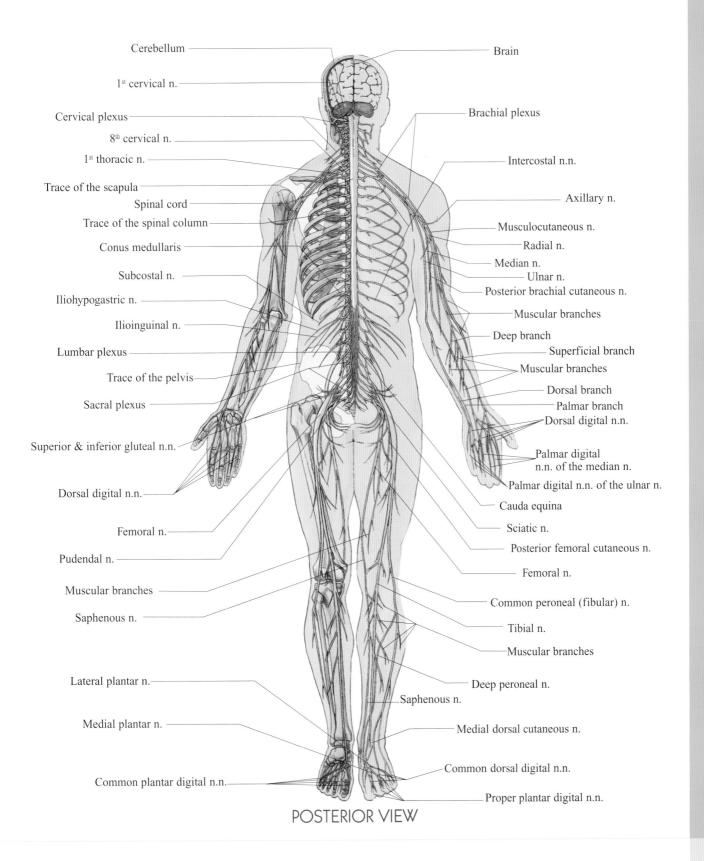

Cerebellum

Brain

1ˢᵗ cervical n.

Cervical plexus

Brachial plexus

8ᵗʰ cervical n.

1ˢᵗ thoracic n.

Intercostal n.n.

Trace of the scapula

Spinal cord

Axillary n.

Trace of the spinal column

Musculocutaneous n.

Conus medullaris

Radial n.

Median n.

Subcostal n.

Ulnar n.

Iliohypogastric n.

Posterior brachial cutaneous n.

Ilioinguinal n.

Muscular branches

Deep branch

Lumbar plexus

Superficial branch

Trace of the pelvis

Muscular branches

Sacral plexus

Dorsal branch

Palmar branch

Dorsal digital n.n.

Superior & inferior gluteal n.n.

Palmar digital
n.n. of the median n.

Dorsal digital n.n.

Palmar digital n.n. of the ulnar n.

Cauda equina

Femoral n.

Sciatic n.

Pudendal n.

Posterior femoral cutaneous n.

Muscular branches

Femoral n.

Saphenous n.

Common peroneal (fibular) n.

Tibial n.

Muscular branches

Lateral plantar n.

Deep peroneal n.

Saphenous n.

Medial plantar n.

Medial dorsal cutaneous n.

Common dorsal digital n.n.

Common plantar digital n.n.

Proper plantar digital n.n.

POSTERIOR VIEW

CUTANEOUS INNERVATION
DERMATOMES & PERIPHERAL NERVE DISTRIBUTIONS

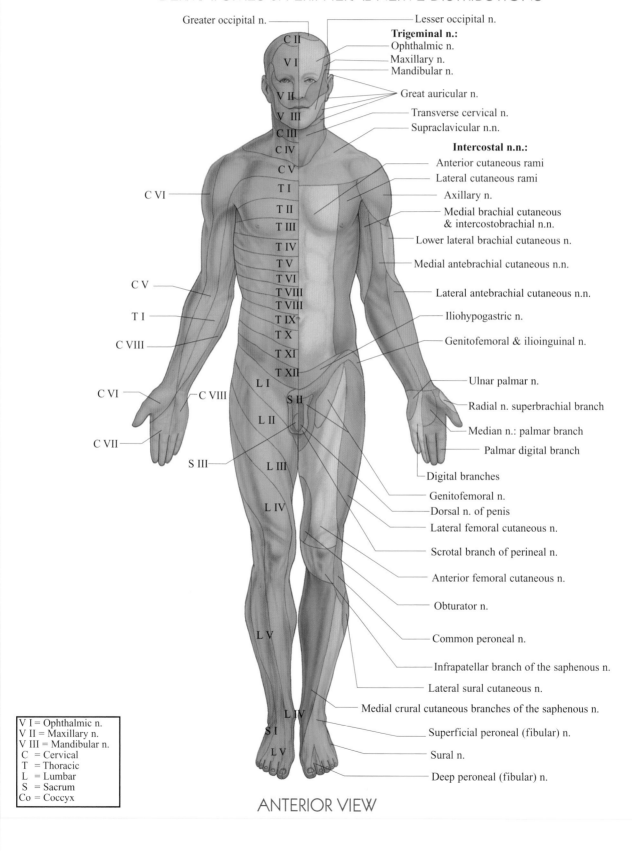

Greater occipital n.

Lesser occipital n.

Trigeminal n.:
Ophthalmic n.
Maxillary n.
Mandibular n.

Great auricular n.

Transverse cervical n.

Supraclavicular n.n.

Intercostal n.n.:

Anterior cutaneous rami

Lateral cutaneous rami

Axillary n.

Medial brachial cutaneous
& intercostobrachial n.n.

Lower lateral brachial cutaneous n.

Medial antebrachial cutaneous n.n.

Lateral antebrachial cutaneous n.n.

Iliohypogastric n.

Genitofemoral & ilioinguinal n.

Ulnar palmar n.

Radial n. superbrachial branch

Median n.: palmar branch

Palmar digital branch

Digital branches

Genitofemoral n.

Dorsal n. of penis

Lateral femoral cutaneous n.

Scrotal branch of perineal n.

Anterior femoral cutaneous n.

Obturator n.

Common peroneal n.

Infrapatellar branch of the saphenous n.

Lateral sural cutaneous n.

Medial crural cutaneous branches of the saphenous n.

Superficial peroneal (fibular) n.

Sural n.

Deep peroneal (fibular) n.

C II
V I
V II
V III
C III
C IV
C V
T I
T II
T III
T IV
T V
T VI
T VII
T VIII
T IX
T X
T XI
T XII
L I
S II
L II
L III
L IV
L V
L IV
S I
L V

C VI
C V
T I
C VIII
C VI
C VII
C VIII
S III

V I = Ophthalmic n.
V II = Maxillary n.
V III = Mandibular n.
C = Cervical
T = Thoracic
L = Lumbar
S = Sacrum
Co = Coccyx

ANTERIOR VIEW

CUTANEOUS INNERVATION
DERMATOMES & PERIPHERAL NERVE DISTRIBUTIONS

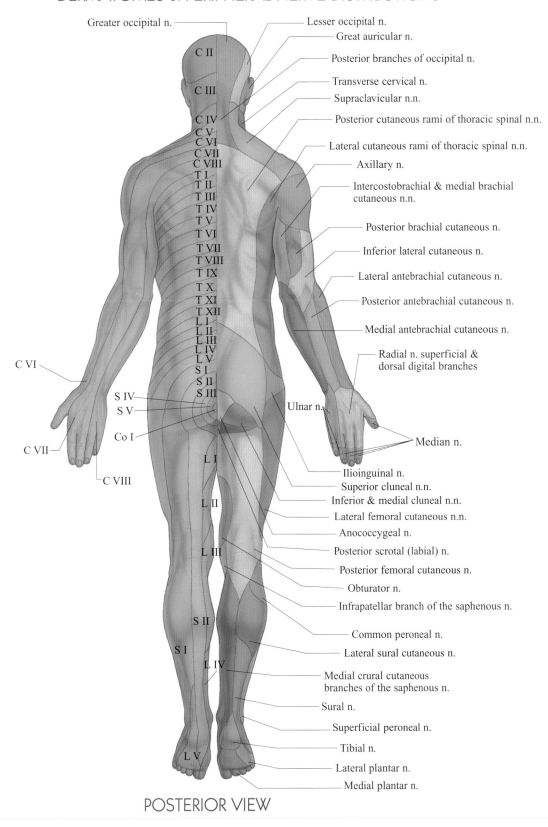

Greater occipital n.

Lesser occipital n.

Great auricular n.

Posterior branches of occipital n.

Transverse cervical n.

Supraclavicular n.n.

Posterior cutaneous rami of thoracic spinal n.n.

Lateral cutaneous rami of thoracic spinal n.n.

Axillary n.

Intercostobrachial & medial brachial cutaneous n.n.

Posterior brachial cutaneous n.

Inferior lateral cutaneous n.

Lateral antebrachial cutaneous n.

Posterior antebrachial cutaneous n.

Medial antebrachial cutaneous n.

Radial n. superficial & dorsal digital branches

Ulnar n.

Median n.

Ilioinguinal n.

Superior cluneal n.n.

Inferior & medial cluneal n.n.

Lateral femoral cutaneous n.n.

Anococcygeal n.

Posterior scrotal (labial) n.

Posterior femoral cutaneous n.

Obturator n.

Infrapatellar branch of the saphenous n.

Common peroneal n.

Lateral sural cutaneous n.

Medial crural cutaneous branches of the saphenous n.

Sural n.

Superficial peroneal n.

Tibial n.

Lateral plantar n.

Medial plantar n.

C II
C III
C IV
C V
C VI
C VII
C VIII
T I
T II
T III
T IV
T V
T VI
T VII
T VIII
T IX
T X
T XI
T XII
L I
L II
L III
L IV
L V
S I
S II
S III
S IV
S V
Co I

C VI
C VII
C VIII

L I
L II
L III
S II
S I
L IV
L V

POSTERIOR VIEW

105

CERVICOBRACHIAL PLEXUS

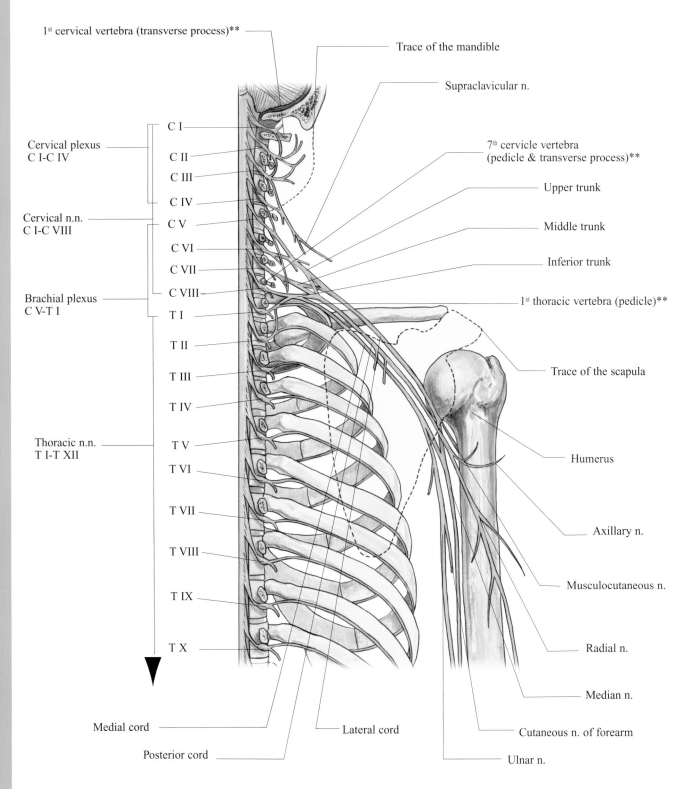

1st cervical vertebra (transverse process)**

Trace of the mandible

Supraclavicular n.

Cervical plexus
C I-C IV

C I

C II

C III

C IV

7th cervicle vertebra
(pedicle & transverse process)**

Upper trunk

Cervical n.n.
C I-C VIII

C V

C VI

C VII

C VIII

Middle trunk

Inferior trunk

Brachial plexus
C V-T I

T I

1st thoracic vertebra (pedicle)**

Trace of the scapula

T II

T III

T IV

Thoracic n.n.
T I-T XII

T V

Humerus

T VI

T VII

T VIII

Axillary n.

T IX

Musculocutaneous n.

T X

Radial n.

Median n.

Medial cord

Lateral cord

Cutaneous n. of forearm

Posterior cord

Ulnar n.

POSTERIOR VIEW

LUMBOSACRAL PLEXUS

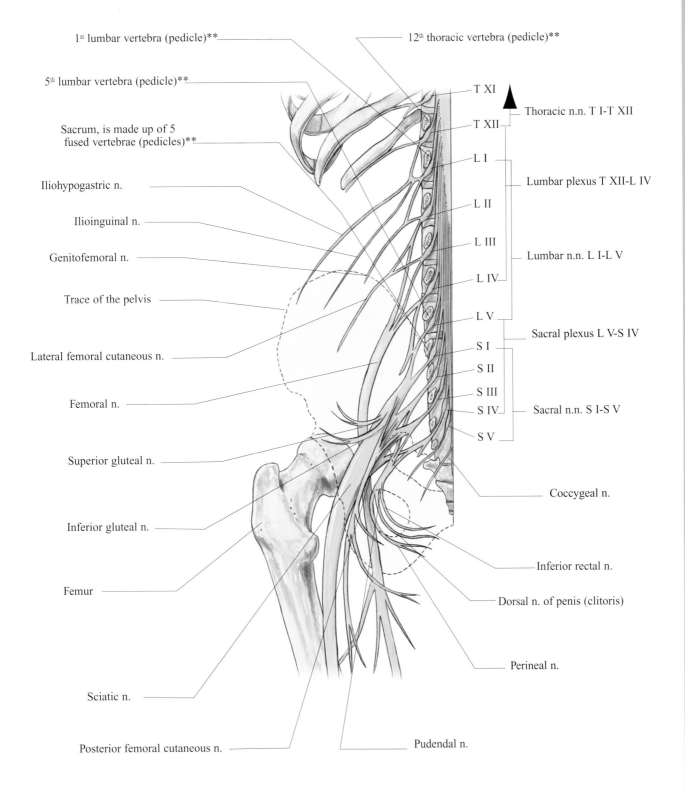

1st lumbar vertebra (pedicle)**

12th thoracic vertebra (pedicle)**

5th lumbar vertebra (pedicle)**

T XI

Thoracic n.n. T I-T XII

T XII

Sacrum, is made up of 5
fused vertebrae (pedicles)**

L I

Lumbar plexus T XII-L IV

L II

Iliohypogastric n.

L III

Ilioinguinal n.

Lumbar n.n. L I-L V

Genitofemoral n.

L IV

Trace of the pelvis

L V

Lateral femoral cutaneous n.

S I

Sacral plexus L V-S IV

S II

S III

Femoral n.

S IV

Sacral n.n. S I-S V

S V

Superior gluteal n.

Coccygeal n.

Inferior gluteal n.

Inferior rectal n.

Femur

Dorsal n. of penis (clitoris)

Perineal n.

Sciatic n.

Posterior femoral cutaneous n.

Pudendal n.

POSTERIOR VIEW

SPINAL CORD

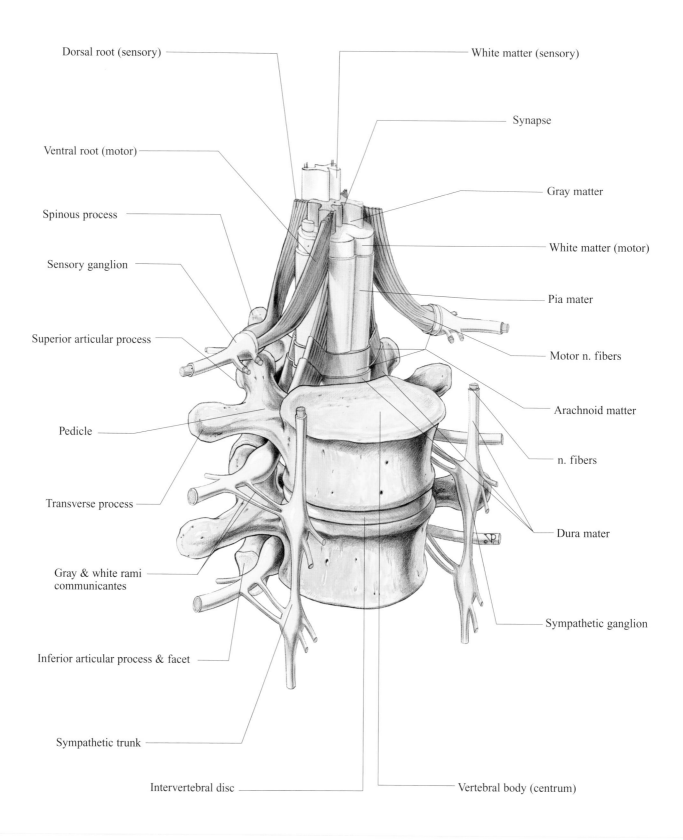

Dorsal root (sensory)

White matter (sensory)

Synapse

Ventral root (motor)

Gray matter

Spinous process

White matter (motor)

Sensory ganglion

Pia mater

Superior articular process

Motor n. fibers

Pedicle

Arachnoid matter

n. fibers

Transverse process

Dura mater

Gray & white rami
communicantes

Sympathetic ganglion

Inferior articular process & facet

Sympathetic trunk

Intervertebral disc

Vertebral body (centrum)

SCIATIC NERVE

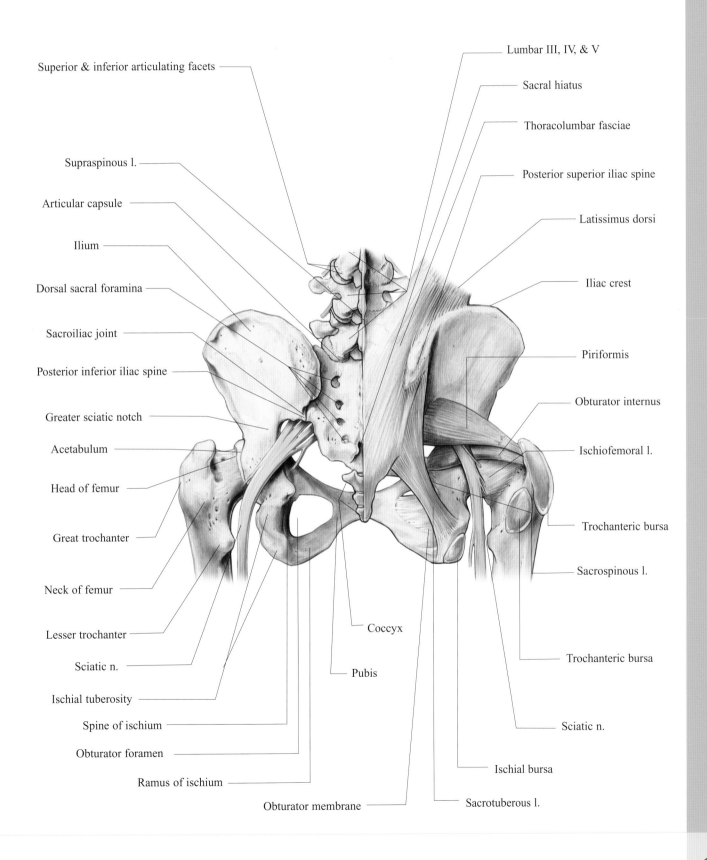

Superior & inferior articulating facets

Supraspinous l.

Articular capsule

Ilium

Dorsal sacral foramina

Sacroiliac joint

Posterior inferior iliac spine

Greater sciatic notch

Acetabulum

Head of femur

Great trochanter

Neck of femur

Lesser trochanter

Sciatic n.

Ischial tuberosity

Spine of ischium

Obturator foramen

Ramus of ischium

Obturator membrane

Coccyx

Pubis

Sacrotuberous l.

Lumbar III, IV, & V

Sacral hiatus

Thoracolumbar fasciae

Posterior superior iliac spine

Latissimus dorsi

Iliac crest

Piriformis

Obturator internus

Ischiofemoral l.

Trochanteric bursa

Sacrospinous l.

Trochanteric bursa

Sciatic n.

Ischial bursa

TRIGEMINAL NERVE

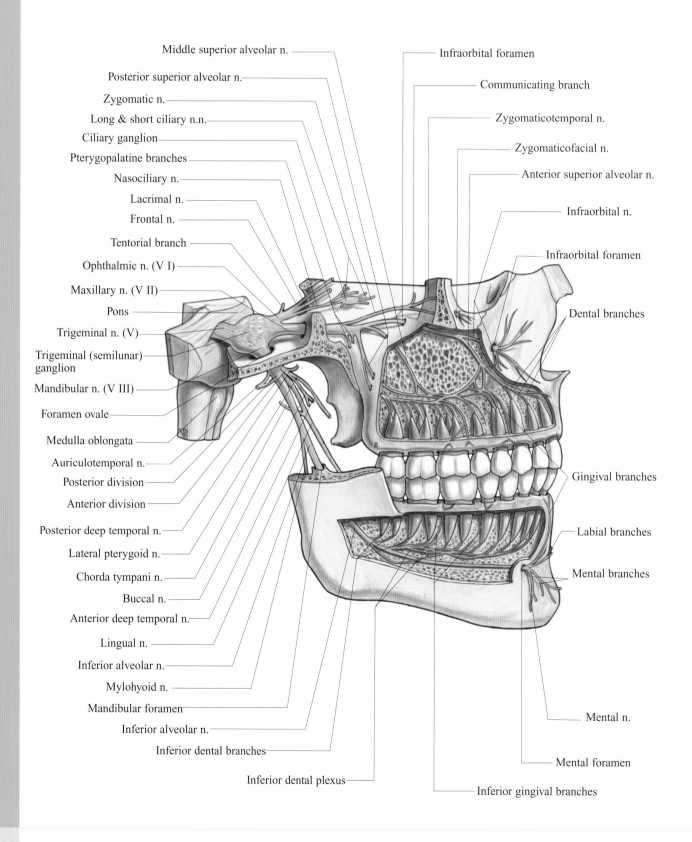

Middle superior alveolar n.

Posterior superior alveolar n.

Zygomatic n.

Long & short ciliary n.n.

Ciliary ganglion

Pterygopalatine branches

Nasociliary n.

Lacrimal n.

Frontal n.

Tentorial branch

Ophthalmic n. (V I)

Maxillary n. (V II)

Pons

Trigeminal n. (V)

Trigeminal (semilunar) ganglion

Mandibular n. (V III)

Foramen ovale

Medulla oblongata

Auriculotemporal n.

Posterior division

Anterior division

Posterior deep temporal n.

Lateral pterygoid n.

Chorda tympani n.

Buccal n.

Anterior deep temporal n.

Lingual n.

Inferior alveolar n.

Mylohyoid n.

Mandibular foramen

Inferior alveolar n.

Inferior dental branches

Inferior dental plexus

Infraorbital foramen

Communicating branch

Zygomaticotemporal n.

Zygomaticofacial n.

Anterior superior alveolar n.

Infraorbital n.

Infraorbital foramen

Dental branches

Gingival branches

Labial branches

Mental branches

Mental n.

Mental foramen

Inferior gingival branches

NERVES OF THE FACE & HEAD

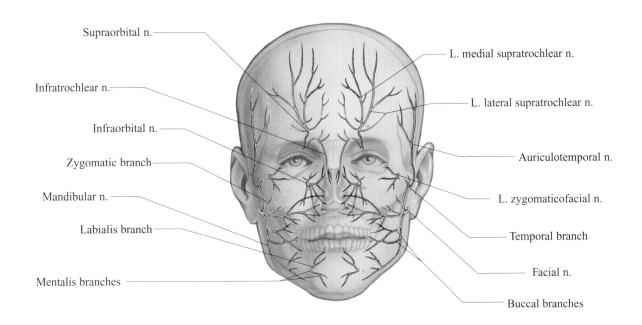

Supraorbital n.

Infratrochlear n.

Infraorbital n.

Zygomatic branch

Mandibular n.

Labialis branch

Mentalis branches

L. medial supratrochlear n.

L. lateral supratrochlear n.

Auriculotemporal n.

L. zygomaticofacial n.

Temporal branch

Facial n.

Buccal branches

NERVE STRUCTURE

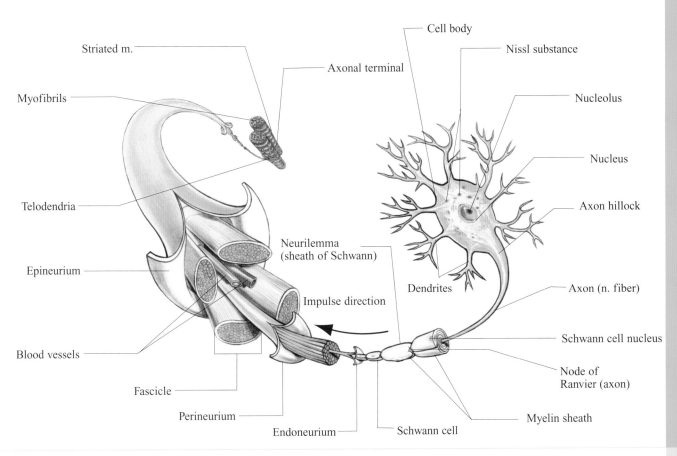

Striated m.

Myofibrils

Telodendria

Epineurium

Blood vessels

Fascicle

Perineurium

Endoneurium

Axonal terminal

Neurilemma
(sheath of Schwann)

Impulse direction

Schwann cell

Cell body

Nissl substance

Nucleolus

Nucleus

Axon hillock

Dendrites

Axon (n. fiber)

Schwann cell nucleus

Node of
Ranvier (axon)

Myelin sheath

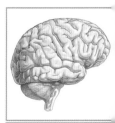

7

THE BRAIN

BRAIN IN PLACE

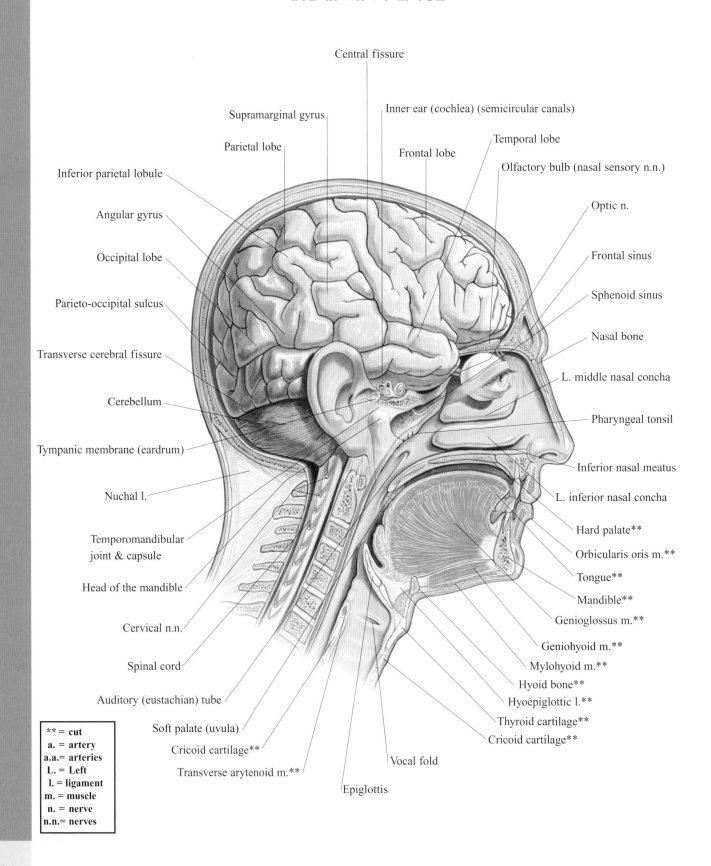

Central fissure

Supramarginal gyrus

Parietal lobe

Inferior parietal lobule

Angular gyrus

Occipital lobe

Parieto-occipital sulcus

Transverse cerebral fissure

Cerebellum

Tympanic membrane (eardrum)

Nuchal l.

Temporomandibular joint & capsule

Head of the mandible

Cervical n.n.

Spinal cord

Auditory (eustachian) tube

Soft palate (uvula)

Cricoid cartilage**

Transverse arytenoid m.**

Inner ear (cochlea) (semicircular canals)

Frontal lobe

Temporal lobe

Olfactory bulb (nasal sensory n.n.)

Optic n.

Frontal sinus

Sphenoid sinus

Nasal bone

L. middle nasal concha

Pharyngeal tonsil

Inferior nasal meatus

L. inferior nasal concha

Hard palate**

Orbicularis oris m.**

Tongue**

Mandible**

Genioglossus m.**

Geniohyoid m.**

Mylohyoid m.**

Hyoid bone**

Hyoepiglottic l.**

Thyroid cartilage**

Cricoid cartilage**

Vocal fold

Epiglottis

** = cut
a. = artery
a.a.= arteries
L. = Left
l. = ligament
m. = muscle
n. = nerve
n.n.= nerves

BRAIN

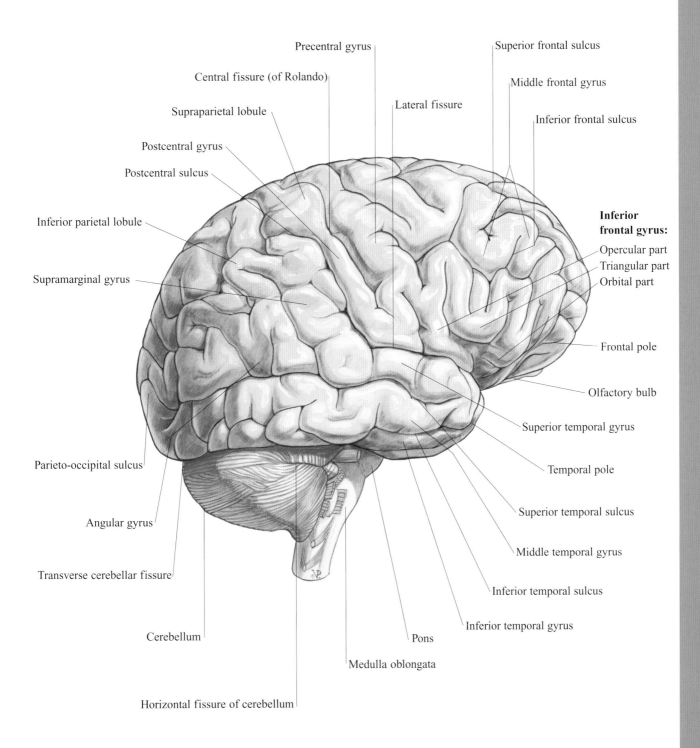

Precentral gyrus

Central fissure (of Rolando)

Supraparietal lobule

Postcentral gyrus

Postcentral sulcus

Inferior parietal lobule

Supramarginal gyrus

Parieto-occipital sulcus

Angular gyrus

Transverse cerebellar fissure

Cerebellum

Horizontal fissure of cerebellum

Superior frontal sulcus

Middle frontal gyrus

Inferior frontal sulcus

Lateral fissure

**Inferior
frontal gyrus:**

Opercular part

Triangular part

Orbital part

Frontal pole

Olfactory bulb

Superior temporal gyrus

Temporal pole

Superior temporal sulcus

Middle temporal gyrus

Inferior temporal sulcus

Inferior temporal gyrus

Pons

Medulla oblongata

LATERAL VIEW

BRAIN

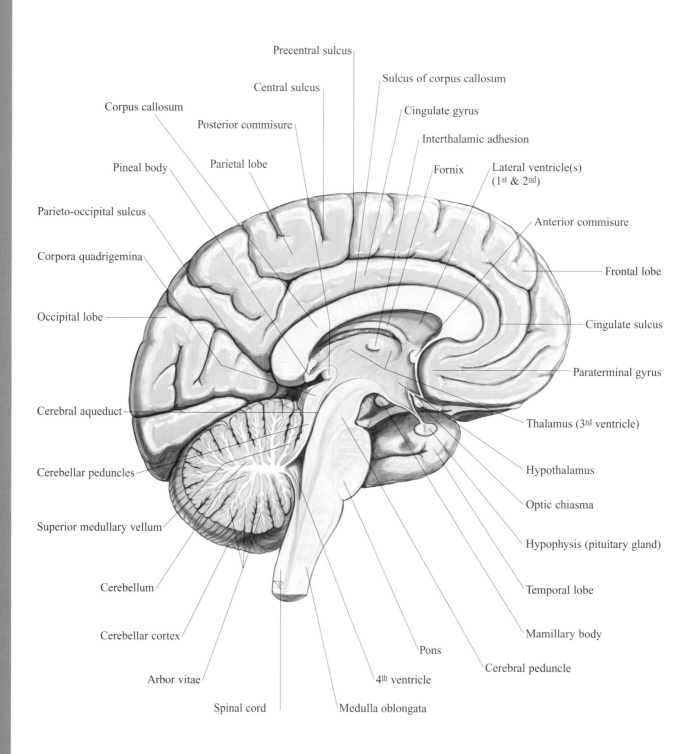

Precentral sulcus

Central sulcus

Sulcus of corpus callosum

Corpus callosum

Posterior commisure

Cingulate gyrus

Interthalamic adhesion

Pineal body

Parietal lobe

Fornix

Lateral ventricle(s)
(1st & 2nd)

Parieto-occipital sulcus

Anterior commisure

Corpora quadrigemina

Frontal lobe

Occipital lobe

Cingulate sulcus

Paraterminal gyrus

Cerebral aqueduct

Thalamus (3rd ventricle)

Hypothalamus

Cerebellar peduncles

Optic chiasma

Superior medullary vellum

Hypophysis (pituitary gland)

Cerebellum

Temporal lobe

Cerebellar cortex

Mamillary body

Arbor vitae

Cerebral peduncle

Spinal cord

Pons

4th ventricle

Medulla oblongata

MEDIAL (SAGITTAL) VIEW

BRAIN

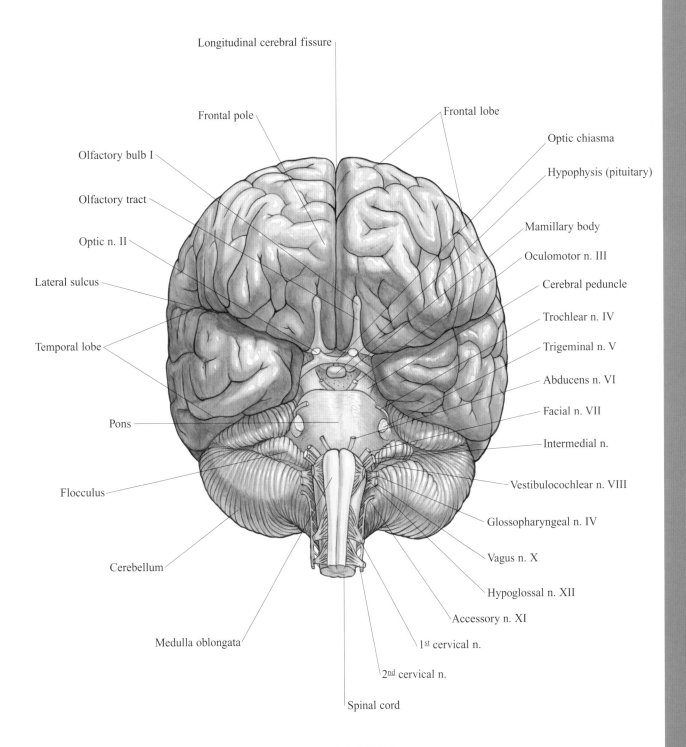

Longitudinal cerebral fissure

Frontal pole

Frontal lobe

Optic chiasma

Olfactory bulb I

Hypophysis (pituitary)

Olfactory tract

Mamillary body

Optic n. II

Oculomotor n. III

Lateral sulcus

Cerebral peduncle

Trochlear n. IV

Temporal lobe

Trigeminal n. V

Abducens n. VI

Pons

Facial n. VII

Intermedial n.

Vestibulocochlear n. VIII

Flocculus

Glossopharyngeal n. IV

Cerebellum

Vagus n. X

Hypoglossal n. XII

Accessory n. XI

Medulla oblongata

1$^{\underline{st}}$ cervical n.

2$^{\underline{nd}}$ cervical n.

Spinal cord

ANTERIOR VIEW

BRAIN

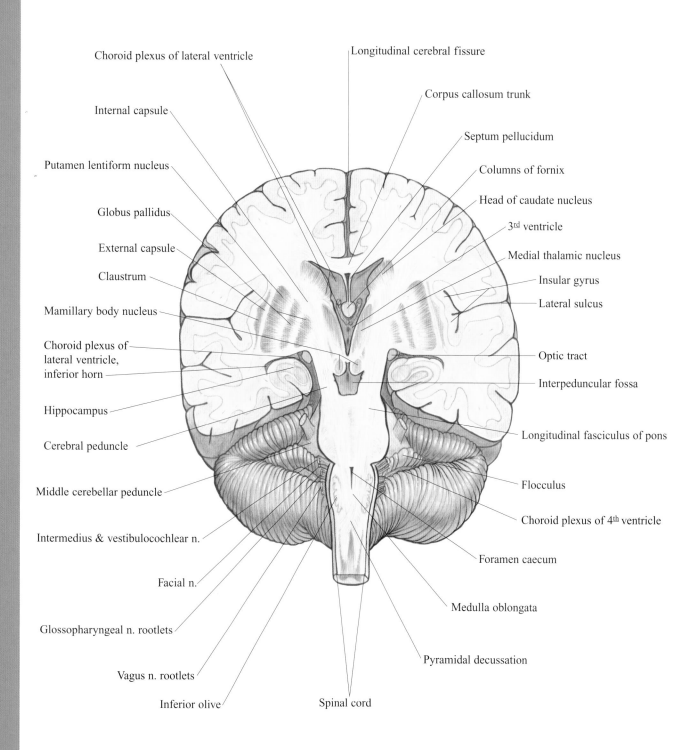

Choroid plexus of lateral ventricle

Internal capsule

Putamen lentiform nucleus

Globus pallidus

External capsule

Claustrum

Mamillary body nucleus

Choroid plexus of
lateral ventricle,
inferior horn

Hippocampus

Cerebral peduncle

Middle cerebellar peduncle

Intermedius & vestibulocochlear n.

Facial n.

Glossopharyngeal n. rootlets

Vagus n. rootlets

Inferior olive

Spinal cord

Longitudinal cerebral fissure

Corpus callosum trunk

Septum pellucidum

Columns of fornix

Head of caudate nucleus

3rd ventricle

Medial thalamic nucleus

Insular gyrus

Lateral sulcus

Optic tract

Interpeduncular fossa

Longitudinal fasciculus of pons

Flocculus

Choroid plexus of 4th ventricle

Foramen caecum

Medulla oblongata

Pyramidal decussation

FRONTAL SECTION

BRAIN

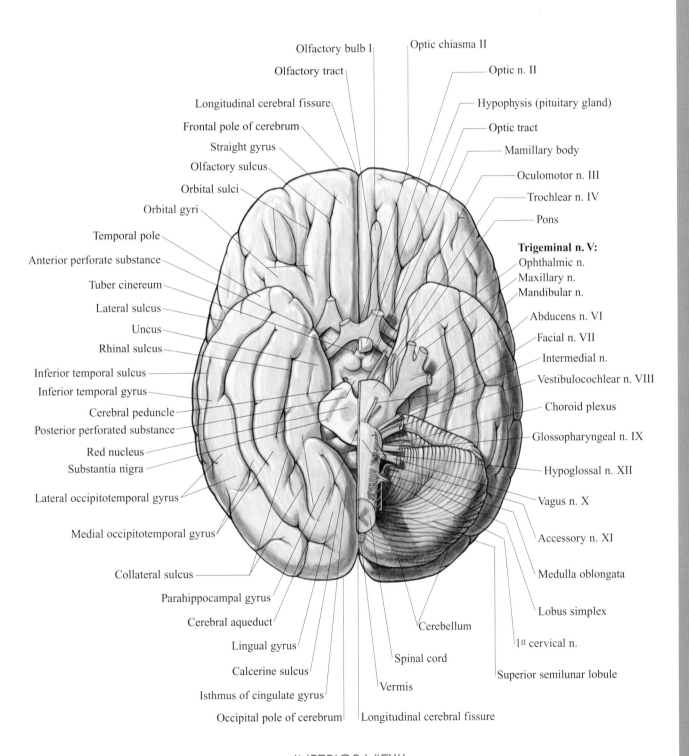

Olfactory bulb I

Olfactory tract

Longitudinal cerebral fissure

Frontal pole of cerebrum

Straight gyrus

Olfactory sulcus

Orbital sulci

Orbital gyri

Temporal pole

Anterior perforate substance

Tuber cinereum

Lateral sulcus

Uncus

Rhinal sulcus

Inferior temporal sulcus

Inferior temporal gyrus

Cerebral peduncle

Posterior perforated substance

Red nucleus

Substantia nigra

Lateral occipitotemporal gyrus

Medial occipitotemporal gyrus

Collateral sulcus

Parahippocampal gyrus

Cerebral aqueduct

Lingual gyrus

Calcerine sulcus

Isthmus of cingulate gyrus

Occipital pole of cerebrum

Optic chiasma II

Optic n. II

Hypophysis (pituitary gland)

Optic tract

Mamillary body

Oculomotor n. III

Trochlear n. IV

Pons

Trigeminal n. V:
Ophthalmic n.
Maxillary n.
Mandibular n.

Abducens n. VI

Facial n. VII

Intermedial n.

Vestibulocochlear n. VIII

Choroid plexus

Glossopharyngeal n. IX

Hypoglossal n. XII

Vagus n. X

Accessory n. XI

Medulla oblongata

Lobus simplex

1ˢᵗ cervical n.

Superior semilunar lobule

Cerebellum

Spinal cord

Vermis

Longitudinal cerebral fissure

INFERIOR VIEW

BRAIN

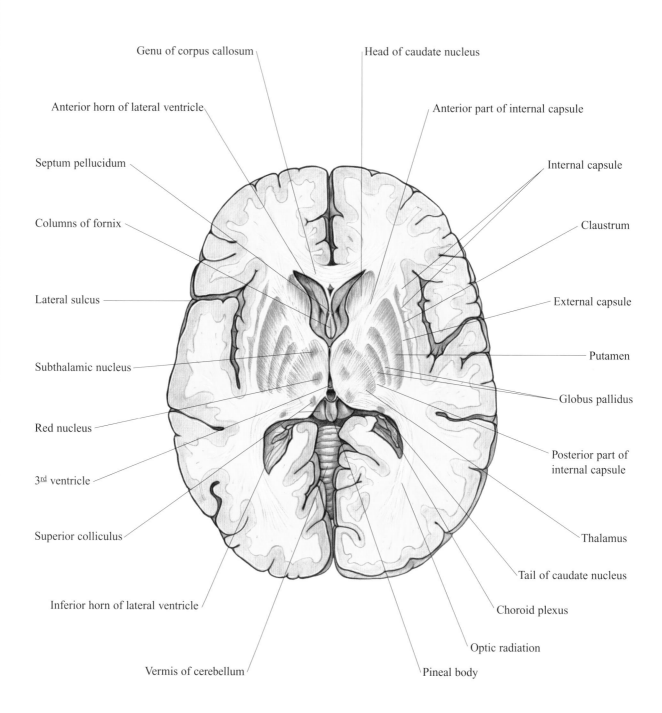

Genu of corpus callosum

Head of caudate nucleus

Anterior horn of lateral ventricle

Anterior part of internal capsule

Septum pellucidum

Internal capsule

Columns of fornix

Claustrum

Lateral sulcus

External capsule

Subthalamic nucleus

Putamen

Red nucleus

Globus pallidus

3rd ventricle

Posterior part of internal capsule

Superior colliculus

Thalamus

Inferior horn of lateral ventricle

Tail of caudate nucleus

Choroid plexus

Optic radiation

Vermis of cerebellum

Pineal body

HORIZONTAL SECTION

BRAIN

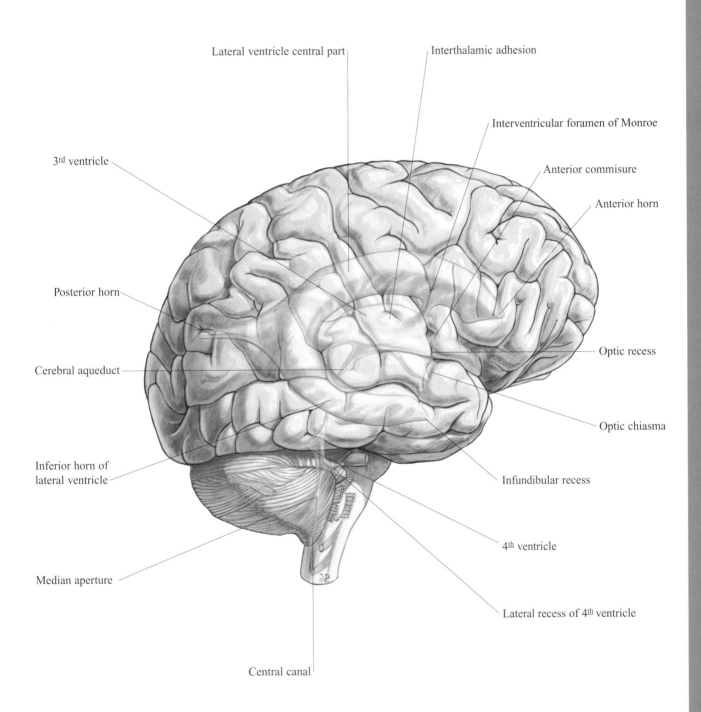

Lateral ventricle central part

Interthalamic adhesion

Interventricular foramen of Monroe

3rd ventricle

Anterior commisure

Anterior horn

Posterior horn

Optic recess

Cerebral aqueduct

Optic chiasma

Inferior horn of
lateral ventricle

Infundibular recess

4th ventricle

Median aperture

Lateral recess of 4th ventricle

Central canal

VENTRICLES

BRAIN

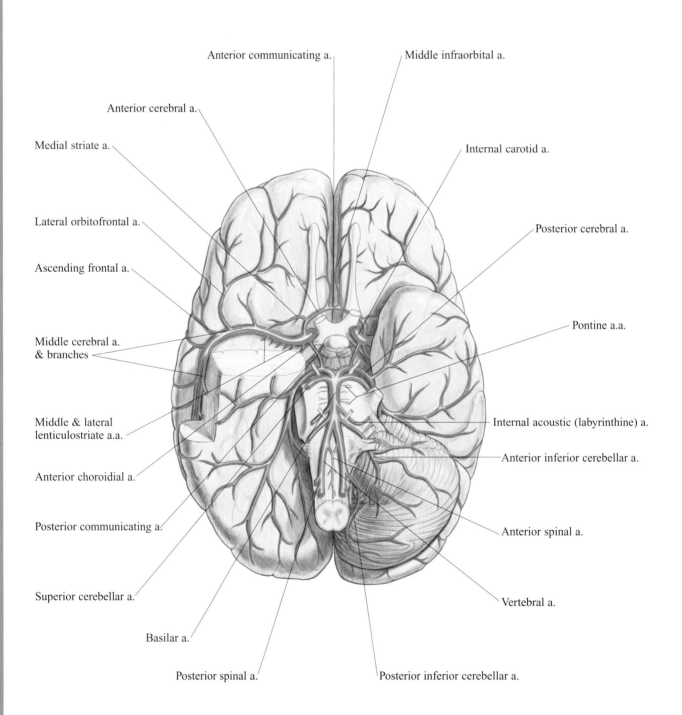

Anterior communicating a.

Middle infraorbital a.

Anterior cerebral a.

Medial striate a.

Internal carotid a.

Lateral orbitofrontal a.

Posterior cerebral a.

Ascending frontal a.

Middle cerebral a.
& branches

Pontine a.a.

Middle & lateral
lenticulostriate a.a.

Internal acoustic (labyrinthine) a.

Anterior inferior cerebellar a.

Anterior choroidial a.

Posterior communicating a.

Anterior spinal a.

Superior cerebellar a.

Vertebral a.

Basilar a.

Posterior spinal a.

Posterior inferior cerebellar a.

ARTERIES

NOTES

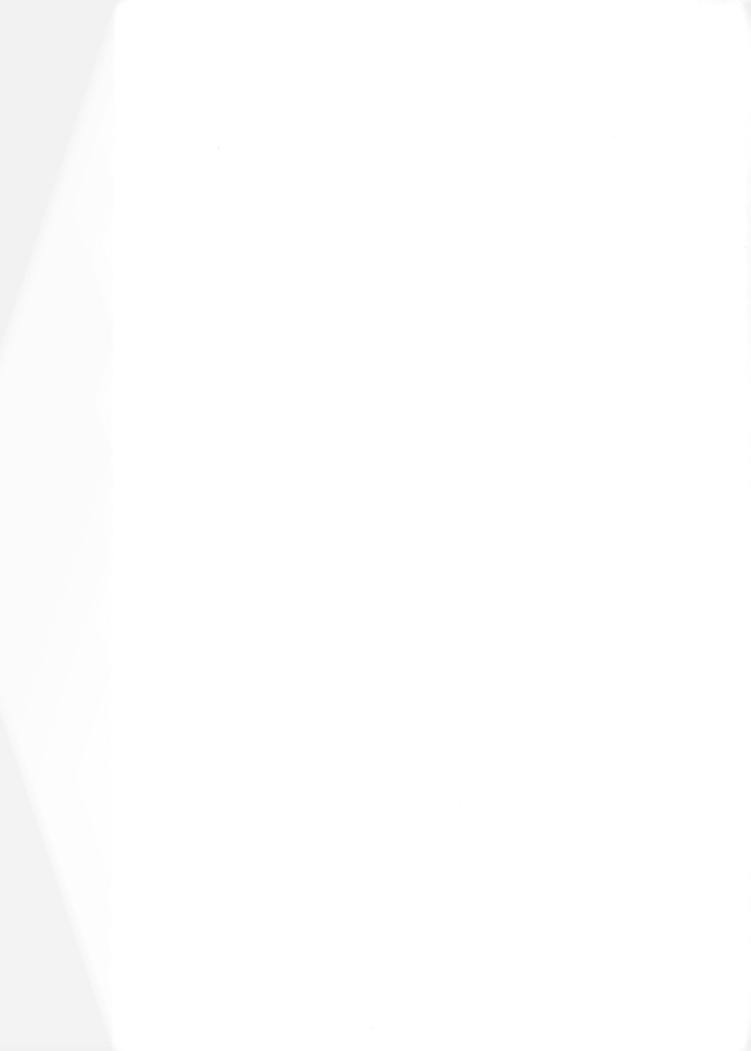

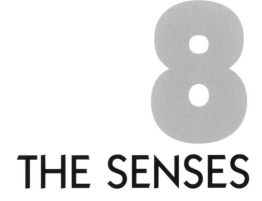

8

THE SENSES

THE SENSES

HEAD: EYE, EAR, NOSE & MOUTH

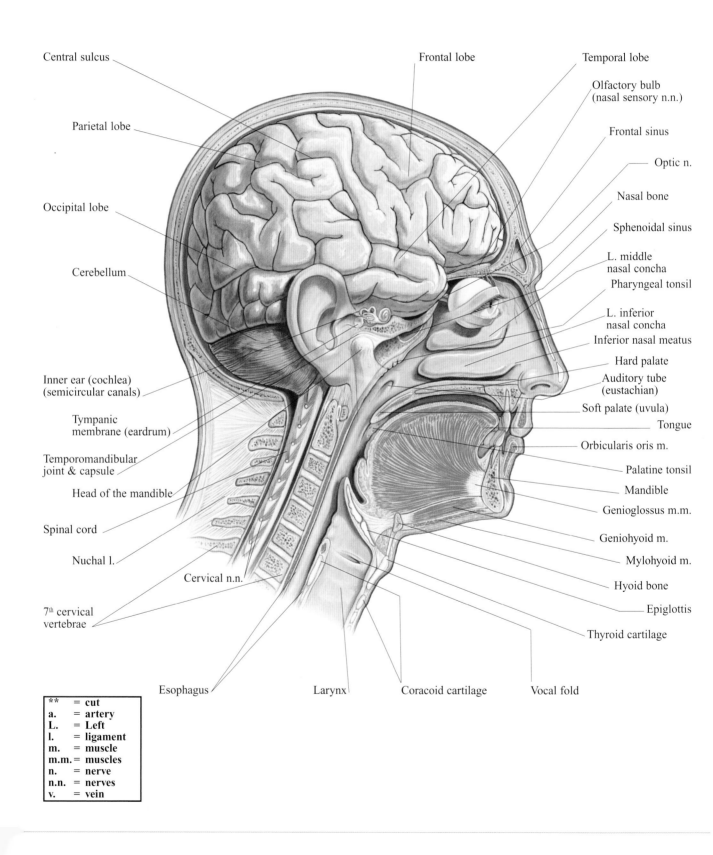

Central sulcus

Frontal lobe

Temporal lobe

Olfactory bulb
(nasal sensory n.n.)

Parietal lobe

Frontal sinus

Optic n.

Nasal bone

Occipital lobe

Sphenoidal sinus

L. middle
nasal concha

Cerebellum

Pharyngeal tonsil

L. inferior
nasal concha

Inferior nasal meatus

Hard palate

Auditory tube
(eustachian)

Inner ear (cochlea)
(semicircular canals)

Soft palate (uvula)

Tongue

Tympanic
membrane (eardrum)

Orbicularis oris m.

Palatine tonsil

Temporomandibular
joint & capsule

Mandible

Head of the mandible

Genioglossus m.m.

Spinal cord

Geniohyoid m.

Nuchal l.

Mylohyoid m.

Cervical n.n.

Hyoid bone

7ᵗʰ cervical
vertebrae

Epiglottis

Thyroid cartilage

Esophagus

Larynx

Coracoid cartilage

Vocal fold

**	= cut
a.	= artery
L.	= Left
l.	= ligament
m.	= muscle
m.m.	= muscles
n.	= nerve
n.n.	= nerves
v.	= vein

SEEING

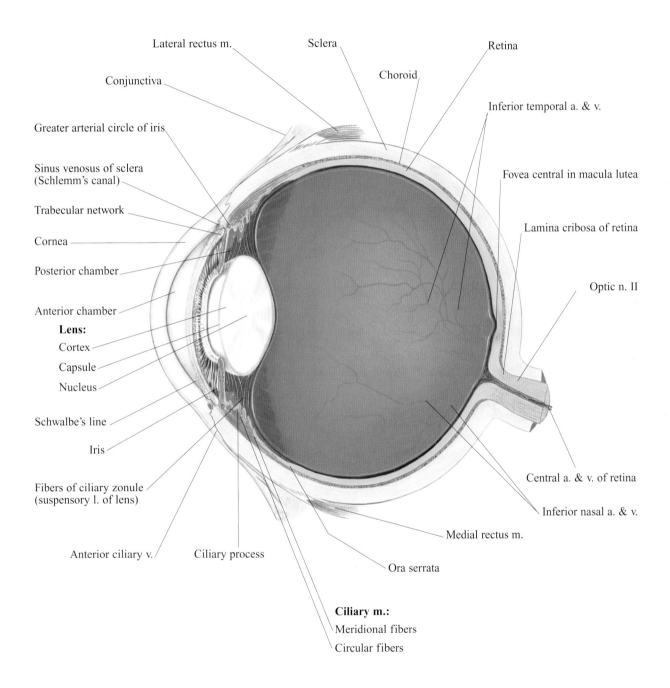

Lateral rectus m.

Conjunctiva

Greater arterial circle of iris

Sinus venosus of sclera
(Schlemm's canal)

Trabecular network

Cornea

Posterior chamber

Anterior chamber

Lens:

Cortex

Capsule

Nucleus

Schwalbe's line

Iris

Fibers of ciliary zonule
(suspensory l. of lens)

Anterior ciliary v.

Ciliary process

Sclera

Choroid

Retina

Inferior temporal a. & v.

Fovea central in macula lutea

Lamina cribosa of retina

Optic n. II

Central a. & v. of retina

Inferior nasal a. & v.

Medial rectus m.

Ora serrata

Ciliary m.:
Meridional fibers
Circular fibers

HEARING

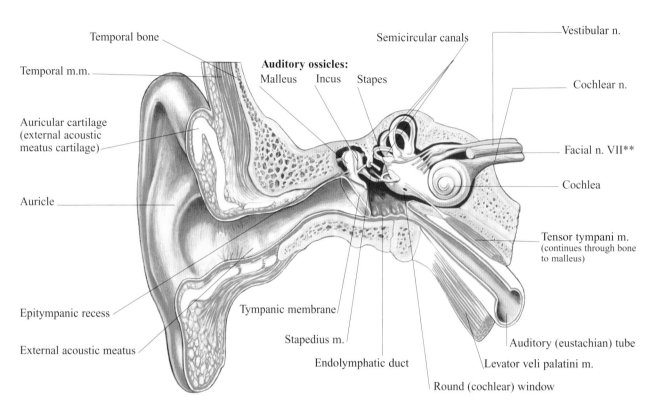

Temporal bone

Temporal m.m.

Auricular cartilage
(external acoustic
meatus cartilage)

Auricle

Epitympanic recess

External acoustic meatus

Auditory ossicles:
Malleus   Incus   Stapes

Semicircular canals

Tympanic membrane

Stapedius m.

Endolymphatic duct

Vestibular n.

Cochlear n.

Facial n. VII**

Cochlea

Tensor tympani m.
(continues through bone
to malleus)

Auditory (eustachian) tube

Levator veli palatini m.

Round (cochlear) window

SEMICIRCULAR CANALS & DUCTS

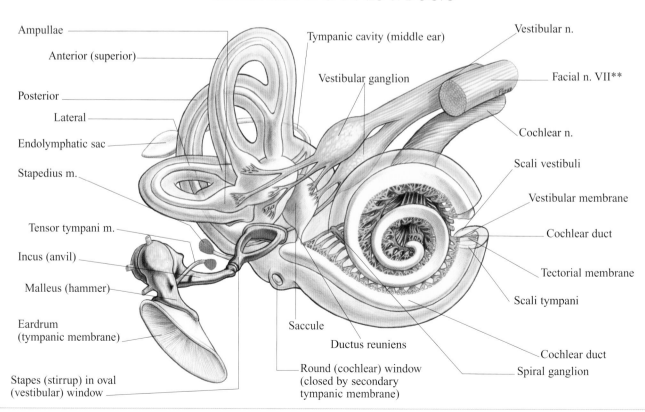

Ampullae

Anterior (superior)

Posterior

Lateral

Endolymphatic sac

Stapedius m.

Tensor tympani m.

Incus (anvil)

Malleus (hammer)

Eardrum
(tympanic membrane)

Stapes (stirrup) in oval
(vestibular) window

Tympanic cavity (middle ear)

Vestibular ganglion

Saccule

Ductus reuniens

Round (cochlear) window
(closed by secondary
tympanic membrane)

Vestibular n.

Facial n. VII**

Cochlear n.

Scali vestibuli

Vestibular membrane

Cochlear duct

Tectorial membrane

Scali tympani

Cochlear duct

Spiral ganglion

SMELL

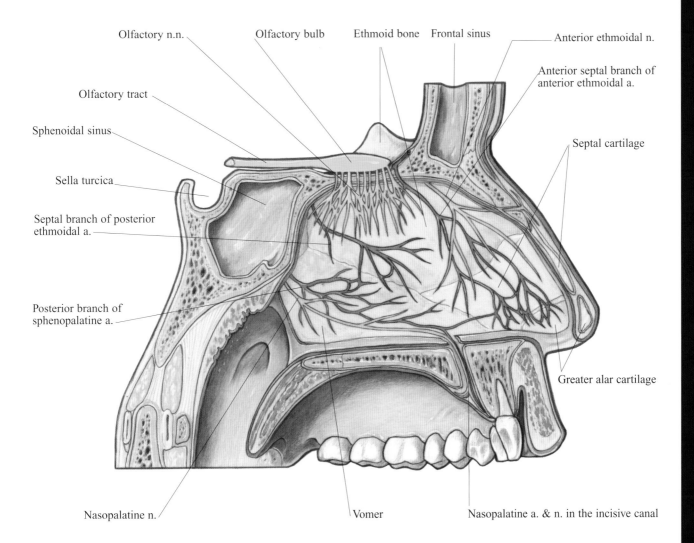

Olfactory n.n.

Olfactory tract

Sphenoidal sinus

Sella turcica

Septal branch of posterior
ethmoidal a.

Posterior branch of
sphenopalatine a.

Nasopalatine n.

Olfactory bulb

Ethmoid bone

Frontal sinus

Anterior ethmoidal n.

Anterior septal branch of
anterior ethmoidal a.

Septal cartilage

Greater alar cartilage

Vomer

Nasopalatine a. & n. in the incisive canal

TASTE

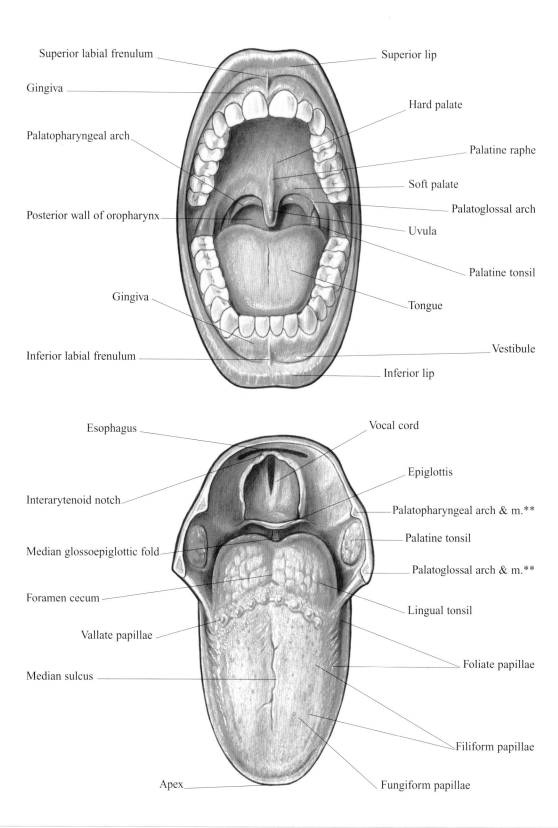

Superior labial frenulum

Superior lip

Gingiva

Hard palate

Palatopharyngeal arch

Palatine raphe

Soft palate

Posterior wall of oropharynx

Palatoglossal arch

Uvula

Palatine tonsil

Gingiva

Tongue

Inferior labial frenulum

Vestibule

Inferior lip

Esophagus

Vocal cord

Epiglottis

Interarytenoid notch

Palatopharyngeal arch & m.**

Palatine tonsil

Median glossoepiglottic fold

Palatoglossal arch & m.**

Foramen cecum

Lingual tonsil

Vallate papillae

Median sulcus

Foliate papillae

Apex

Filiform papillae

Fungiform papillae

TOUCH

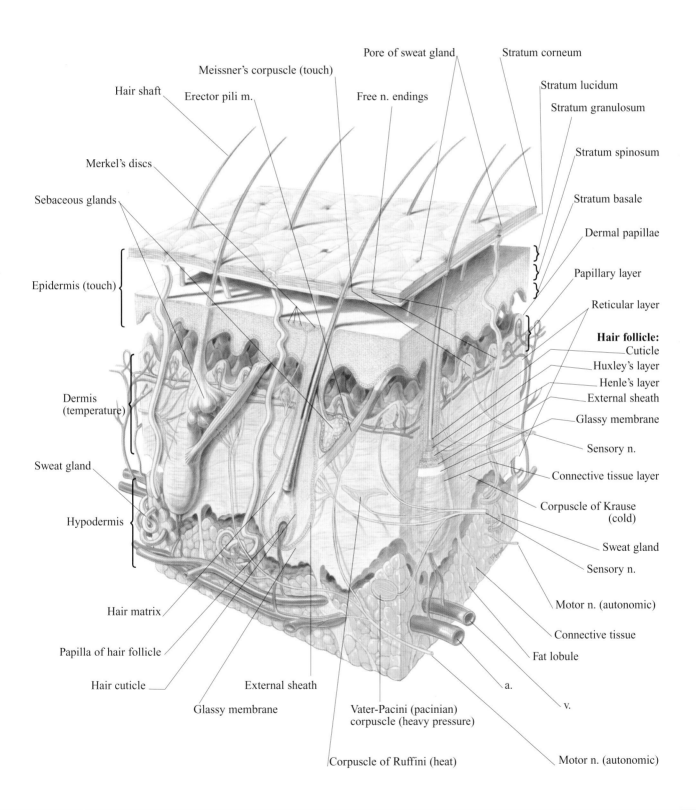

Pore of sweat gland

Stratum corneum

Meissner's corpuscle (touch)

Stratum lucidum

Stratum granulosum

Hair shaft

Erector pili m.

Free n. endings

Stratum spinosum

Merkel's discs

Stratum basale

Dermal papillae

Sebaceous glands

Papillary layer

Epidermis (touch)

Reticular layer

Hair follicle:
Cuticle
Huxley's layer
Henle's layer
External sheath
Glassy membrane
Sensory n.

Dermis
(temperature)

Connective tissue layer

Sweat gland

Corpuscle of Krause
(cold)

Hypodermis

Sweat gland

Sensory n.

Motor n. (autonomic)

Hair matrix

Connective tissue

Papilla of hair follicle

Fat lobule

Hair cuticle

External sheath

a.

Glassy membrane

Vater-Pacini (pacinian)
corpuscle (heavy pressure)

v.

Corpuscle of Ruffini (heat)

Motor n. (autonomic)

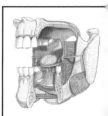

9

DIGESTIVE SYSTEM

DIGESTIVE SYSTEM

DIGESTIVE SYSTEM

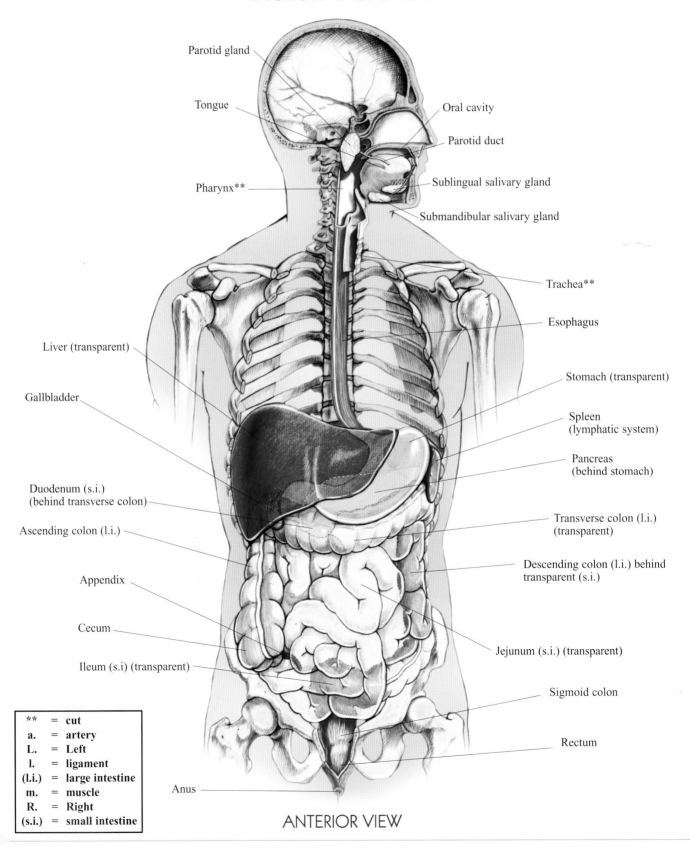

Parotid gland

Tongue

Oral cavity

Parotid duct

Pharynx**

Sublingual salivary gland

Submandibular salivary gland

Trachea**

Esophagus

Liver (transparent)

Stomach (transparent)

Gallbladder

Spleen
(lymphatic system)

Pancreas
(behind stomach)

Duodenum (s.i.)
(behind transverse colon)

Transverse colon (l.i.)
(transparent)

Ascending colon (l.i.)

Descending colon (l.i.) behind
transparent (s.i.)

Appendix

Cecum

Jejunum (s.i.) (transparent)

Ileum (s.i) (transparent)

Sigmoid colon

Rectum

Anus

**	=	cut
a.	=	artery
L.	=	Left
l.	=	ligament
(l.i.)	=	large intestine
m.	=	muscle
R.	=	Right
(s.i.)	=	small intestine

ANTERIOR VIEW

DIGESTIVE SYSTEM

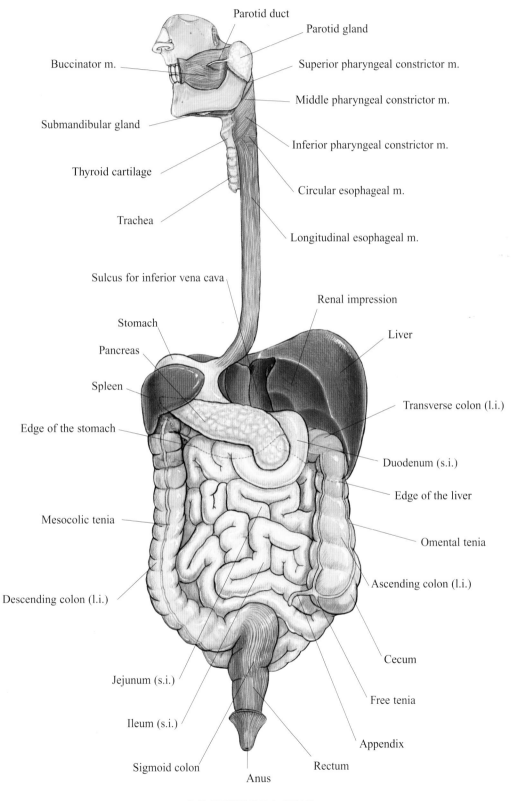

Parotid duct

Parotid gland

Buccinator m.

Superior pharyngeal constrictor m.

Middle pharyngeal constrictor m.

Submandibular gland

Inferior pharyngeal constrictor m.

Thyroid cartilage

Circular esophageal m.

Trachea

Longitudinal esophageal m.

Sulcus for inferior vena cava

Renal impression

Stomach

Liver

Pancreas

Spleen

Transverse colon (l.i.)

Edge of the stomach

Duodenum (s.i.)

Edge of the liver

Mesocolic tenia

Omental tenia

Ascending colon (l.i.)

Descending colon (l.i.)

Cecum

Jejunum (s.i.)

Free tenia

Ileum (s.i.)

Appendix

Sigmoid colon

Rectum

Anus

POSTERIOR VIEW

DIGESTIVE SYSTEM

MOUTH & SALIVARY GLANDS

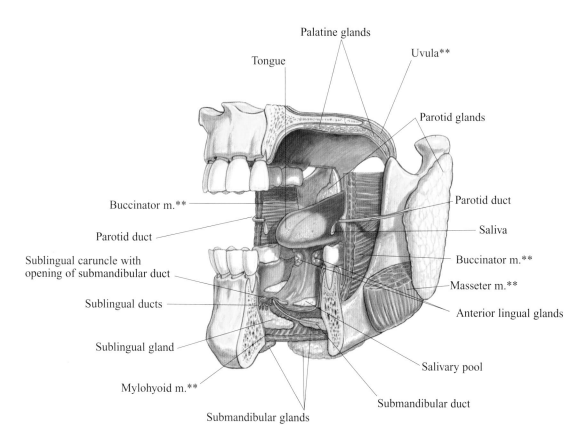

Palatine glands

Tongue

Uvula**

Parotid glands

Buccinator m.**

Parotid duct

Sublingual caruncle with opening of submandibular duct

Sublingual ducts

Sublingual gland

Mylohyoid m.**

Submandibular glands

Parotid duct

Saliva

Buccinator m.**

Masseter m.**

Anterior lingual glands

Salivary pool

Submandibular duct

TONGUE

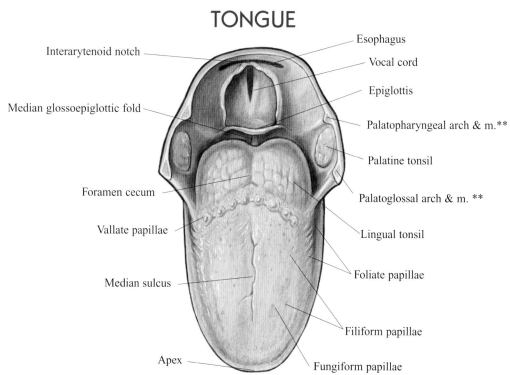

Interarytenoid notch

Median glossoepiglottic fold

Foramen cecum

Vallate papillae

Median sulcus

Apex

Esophagus

Vocal cord

Epiglottis

Palatopharyngeal arch & m.**

Palatine tonsil

Palatoglossal arch & m. **

Lingual tonsil

Foliate papillae

Filiform papillae

Fungiform papillae

STOMACH

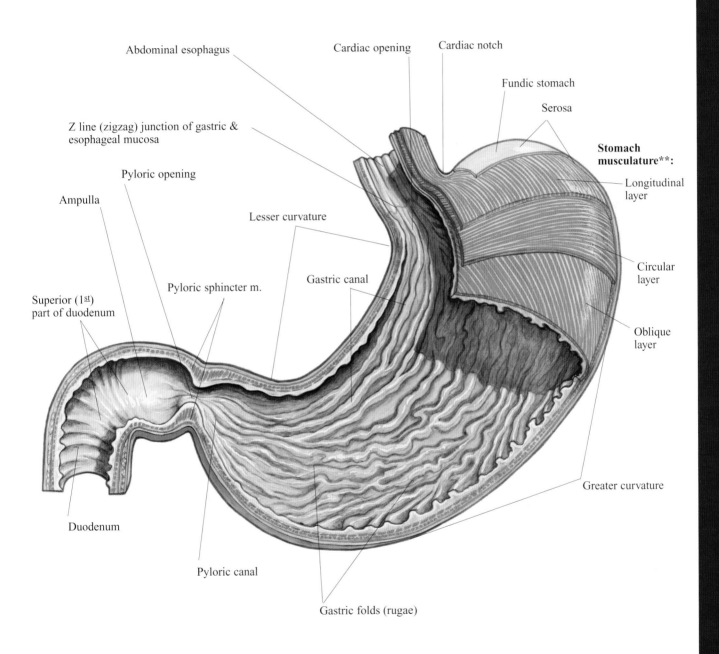

Abdominal esophagus

Cardiac opening

Cardiac notch

Fundic stomach

Serosa

Z line (zigzag) junction of gastric &
esophageal mucosa

**Stomach
musculature**:**

Longitudinal
layer

Pyloric opening

Ampulla

Lesser curvature

Circular
layer

Gastric canal

Superior (1st)
part of duodenum

Pyloric sphincter m.

Oblique
layer

Duodenum

Greater curvature

Pyloric canal

Gastric folds (rugae)

DIGESTIVE SYSTEM

BILE & PANCREATIC DUCT

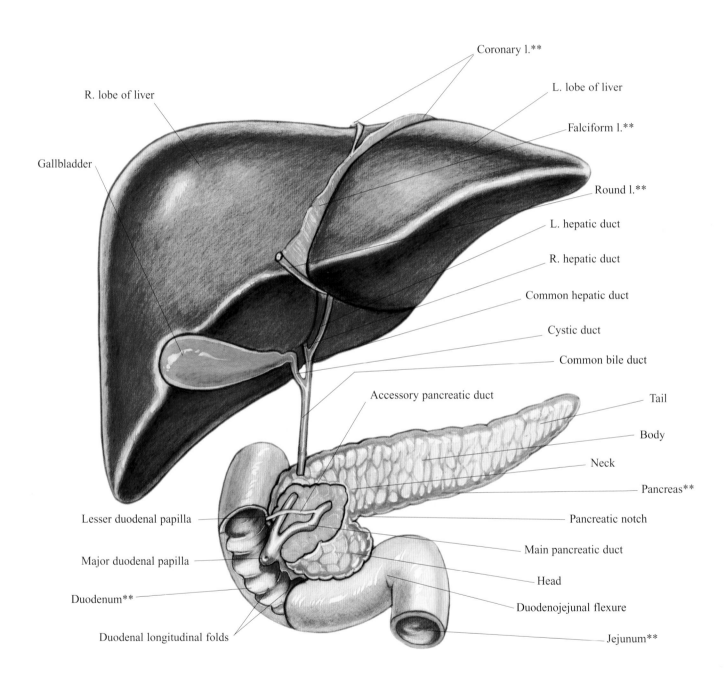

Coronary l.**

L. lobe of liver

Falciform l.**

R. lobe of liver

Round l.**

Gallbladder

L. hepatic duct

R. hepatic duct

Common hepatic duct

Cystic duct

Common bile duct

Accessory pancreatic duct

Tail

Body

Neck

Pancreas**

Lesser duodenal papilla

Pancreatic notch

Main pancreatic duct

Major duodenal papilla

Head

Duodenum**

Duodenojejunal flexure

Duodenal longitudinal folds

Jejunum**

DIGESTIVE SYSTEM

SMALL INTESTINE
(SCHEMATIC)

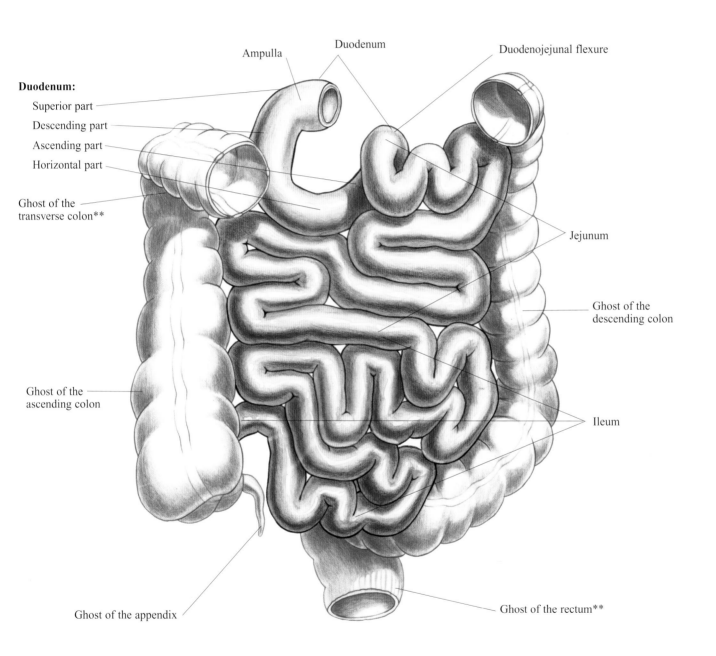

Ampulla

Duodenum

Duodenojejunal flexure

Duodenum:

Superior part

Descending part

Ascending part

Horizontal part

Ghost of the
transverse colon**

Jejunum

Ghost of the
descending colon

Ghost of the
ascending colon

Ileum

Ghost of the appendix

Ghost of the rectum**

DIGESTIVE SYSTEM

LARGE INTESTINE

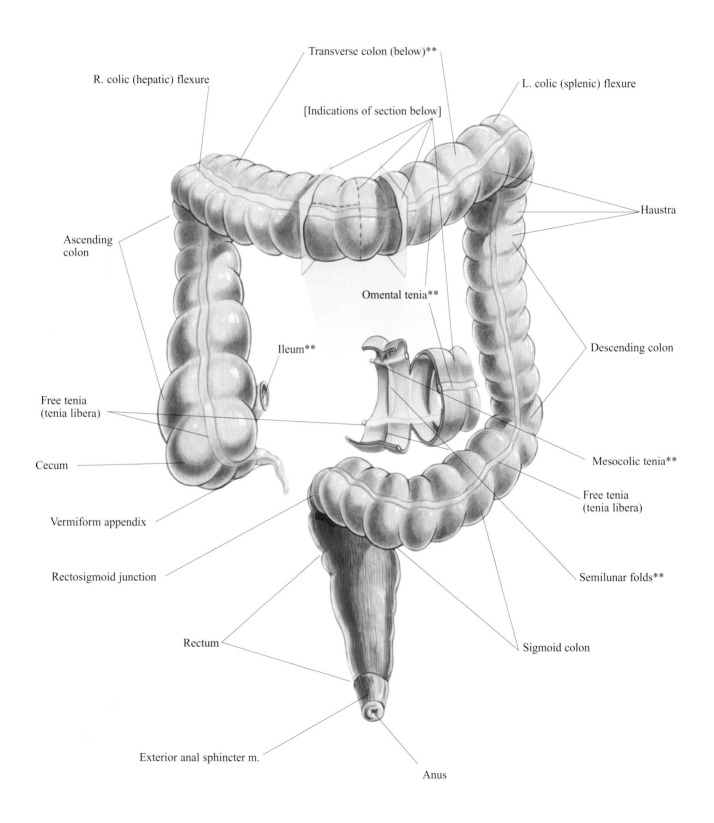

Transverse colon (below)**

R. colic (hepatic) flexure

[Indications of section below]

L. colic (splenic) flexure

Haustra

Ascending
colon

Omental tenia**

Descending colon

Ileum**

Free tenia
(tenia libera)

Cecum

Mesocolic tenia**

Free tenia
(tenia libera)

Vermiform appendix

Rectosigmoid junction

Semilunar folds**

Rectum

Sigmoid colon

Exterior anal sphincter m.

Anus

ILEOCECAL SPHINCTER & APPENDIX

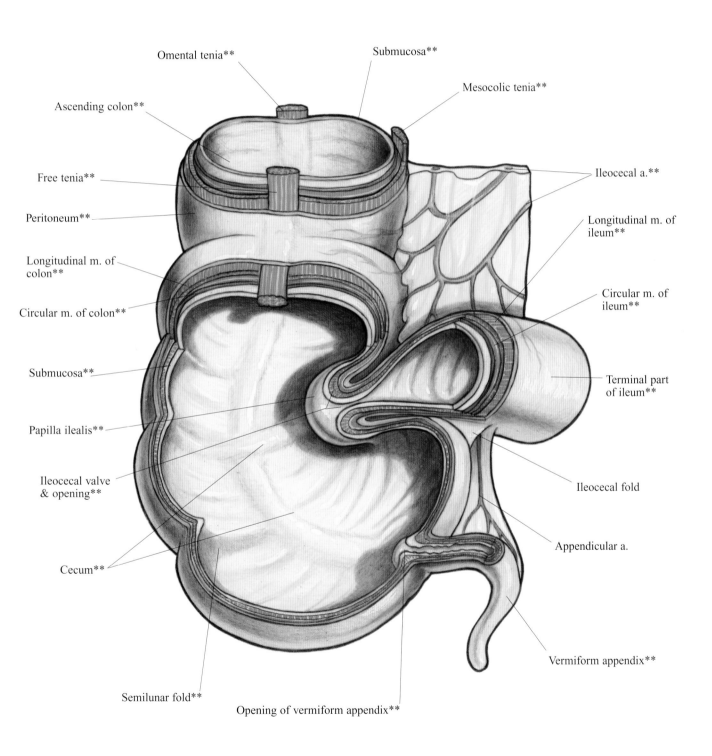

Omental tenia**

Submucosa**

Mesocolic tenia**

Ascending colon**

Free tenia**

Peritoneum**

Longitudinal m. of colon**

Circular m. of colon**

Submucosa**

Papilla ilealis**

Ileocecal valve & opening**

Cecum**

Semilunar fold**

Opening of vermiform appendix**

Ileocecal a.**

Longitudinal m. of ileum**

Circular m. of ileum**

Terminal part of ileum**

Ileocecal fold

Appendicular a.

Vermiform appendix**

RECTUM

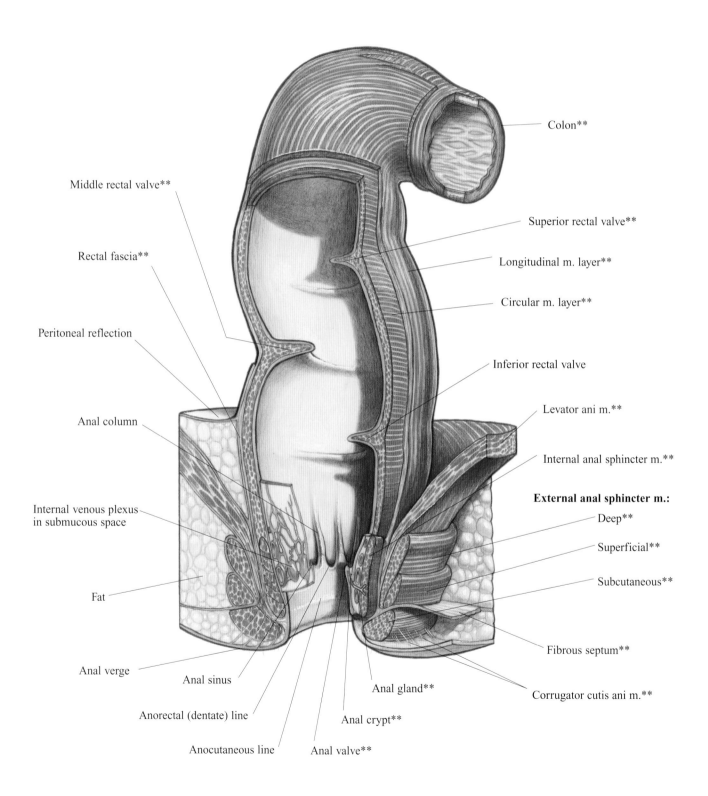

Middle rectal valve**

Rectal fascia**

Peritoneal reflection

Anal column

Internal venous plexus
in submucous space

Fat

Anal verge

Anal sinus

Anorectal (dentate) line

Anocutaneous line

Anal valve**

Anal crypt**

Anal gland**

Colon**

Superior rectal valve**

Longitudinal m. layer**

Circular m. layer**

Inferior rectal valve

Levator ani m.**

Internal anal sphincter m.**

External anal sphincter m.:

Deep**

Superficial**

Subcutaneous**

Fibrous septum**

Corrugator cutis ani m.**

NOTES

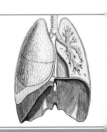

10

RESPIRATORY SYSTEM

RESPIRATORY SYSTEM

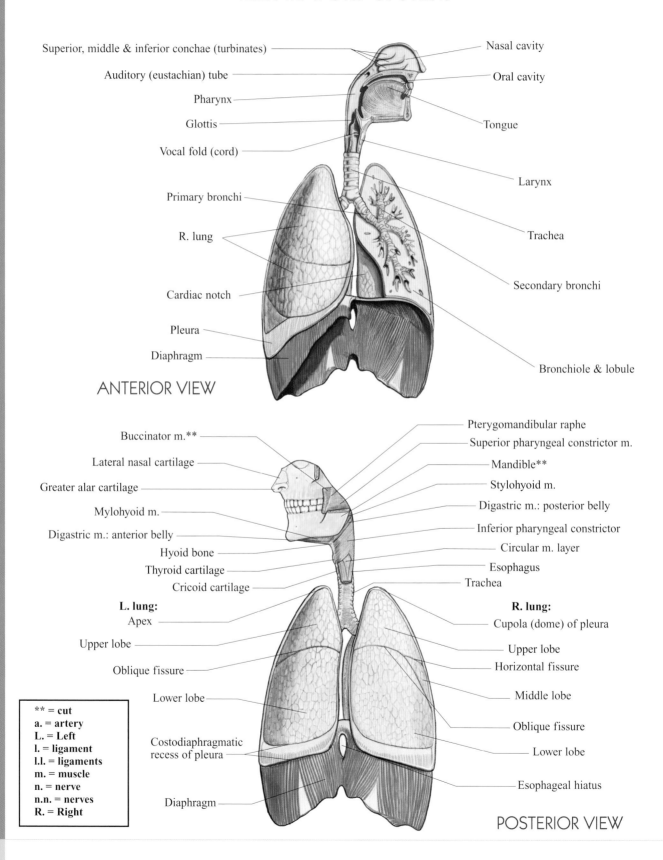

Superior, middle & inferior conchae (turbinates) —

Auditory (eustachian) tube —

Pharynx —

Glottis —

Vocal fold (cord) —

Primary bronchi —

R. lung —

Cardiac notch —

Pleura —

Diaphragm —

Nasal cavity

Oral cavity

Tongue

Larynx

Trachea

Secondary bronchi

Bronchiole & lobule

ANTERIOR VIEW

Buccinator m.** —

Lateral nasal cartilage —

Greater alar cartilage —

Mylohyoid m. —

Digastric m.: anterior belly —

Hyoid bone —

Thyroid cartilage —

Cricoid cartilage —

L. lung:

Apex —

Upper lobe —

Oblique fissure —

Lower lobe —

Costodiaphragmatic recess of pleura —

Diaphragm —

Pterygomandibular raphe

Superior pharyngeal constrictor m.

Mandible**

Stylohyoid m.

Digastric m.: posterior belly

Inferior pharyngeal constrictor

Circular m. layer

Esophagus

Trachea

R. lung:

Cupola (dome) of pleura

Upper lobe

Horizontal fissure

Middle lobe

Oblique fissure

Lower lobe

Esophageal hiatus

** = cut
a. = artery
L. = Left
l. = ligament
l.l. = ligaments
m. = muscle
n. = nerve
n.n. = nerves
R. = Right

POSTERIOR VIEW

146

NASAL & ORAL CAVITY

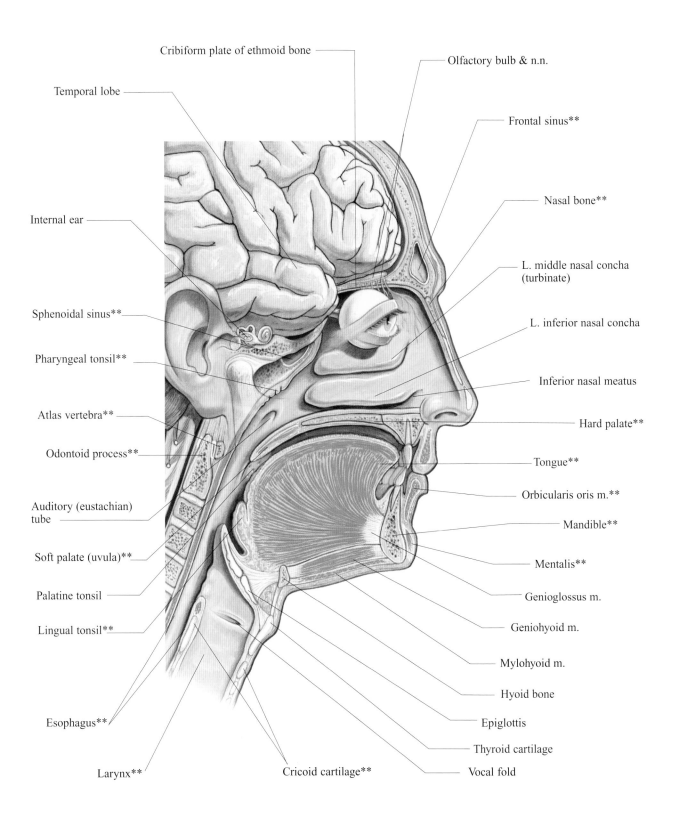

Cribiform plate of ethmoid bone

Olfactory bulb & n.n.

Temporal lobe

Frontal sinus**

Internal ear

Nasal bone**

Sphenoidal sinus**

L. middle nasal concha (turbinate)

Pharyngeal tonsil**

L. inferior nasal concha

Atlas vertebra**

Inferior nasal meatus

Odontoid process**

Hard palate**

Auditory (eustachian) tube

Tongue**

Soft palate (uvula)**

Orbicularis oris m.**

Palatine tonsil

Mandible**

Lingual tonsil**

Mentalis**

Genioglossus m.

Geniohyoid m.

Mylohyoid m.

Esophagus**

Hyoid bone

Epiglottis

Larynx**

Thyroid cartilage

Cricoid cartilage**

Vocal fold

147

NASAL SEPTUM

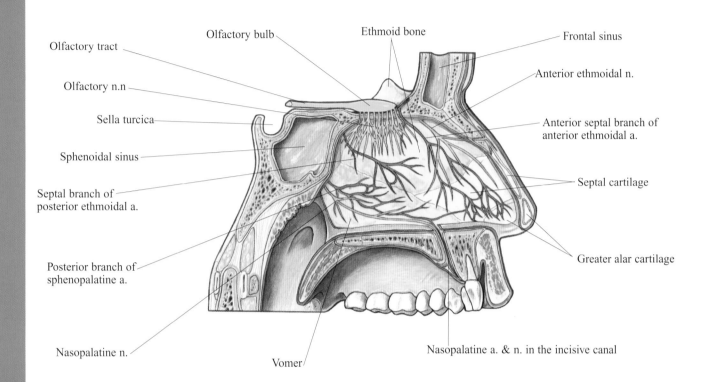

Olfactory tract

Olfactory n.n

Sella turcica

Sphenoidal sinus

Septal branch of
posterior ethmoidal a.

Posterior branch of
sphenopalatine a.

Nasopalatine n.

Olfactory bulb

Ethmoid bone

Frontal sinus

Anterior ethmoidal n.

Anterior septal branch of
anterior ethmoidal a.

Septal cartilage

Greater alar cartilage

Nasopalatine a. & n. in the incisive canal

Vomer

PARANASAL SINUSES

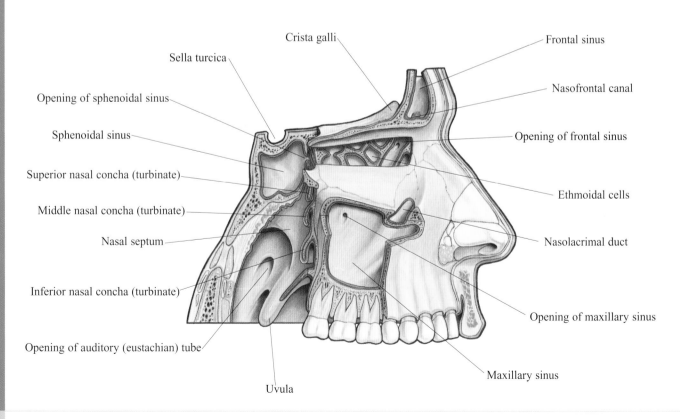

Sella turcica

Crista galli

Frontal sinus

Opening of sphenoidal sinus

Nasofrontal canal

Sphenoidal sinus

Opening of frontal sinus

Superior nasal concha (turbinate)

Ethmoidal cells

Middle nasal concha (turbinate)

Nasal septum

Nasolacrimal duct

Inferior nasal concha (turbinate)

Opening of maxillary sinus

Opening of auditory (eustachian) tube

Maxillary sinus

Uvula

LARYNX

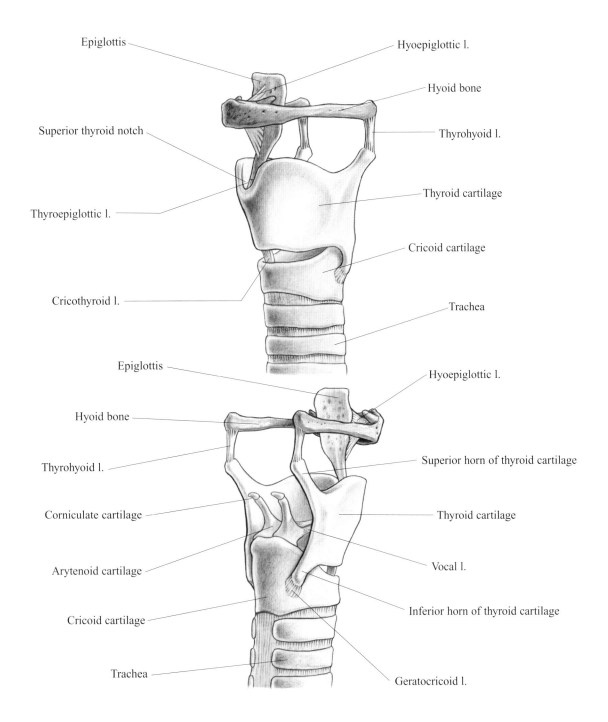

Epiglottis

Hyoepiglottic l.

Hyoid bone

Superior thyroid notch

Thyrohyoid l.

Thyroid cartilage

Thyroepiglottic l.

Cricoid cartilage

Cricothyroid l.

Trachea

Epiglottis

Hyoepiglottic l.

Hyoid bone

Thyrohyoid l.

Superior horn of thyroid cartilage

Corniculate cartilage

Thyroid cartilage

Arytenoid cartilage

Vocal l.

Cricoid cartilage

Inferior horn of thyroid cartilage

Trachea

Geratocricoid l.

BRONCHIAL TREE

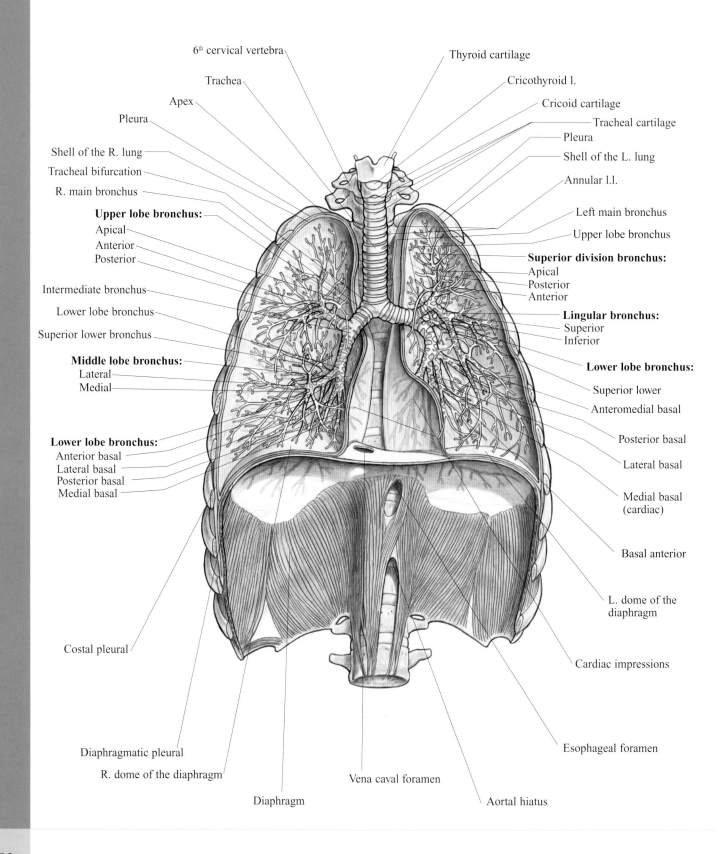

6th cervical vertebra

Trachea

Apex

Pleura

Shell of the R. lung

Tracheal bifurcation

R. main bronchus

Upper lobe bronchus:
Apical
Anterior
Posterior

Intermediate bronchus

Lower lobe bronchus

Superior lower bronchus

Middle lobe bronchus:
Lateral
Medial

Lower lobe bronchus:
Anterior basal
Lateral basal
Posterior basal
Medial basal

Costal pleural

Diaphragmatic pleural

R. dome of the diaphragm

Diaphragm

Thyroid cartilage

Cricothyroid l.

Cricoid cartilage

Tracheal cartilage

Pleura

Shell of the L. lung

Annular l.l.

Left main bronchus

Upper lobe bronchus

Superior division bronchus:
Apical
Posterior
Anterior

Lingular bronchus:
Superior
Inferior

Lower lobe bronchus:

Superior lower

Anteromedial basal

Posterior basal

Lateral basal

Medial basal
(cardiac)

Basal anterior

L. dome of the
diaphragm

Cardiac impressions

Esophageal foramen

Vena caval foramen

Aortal hiatus

MUSCLES OF RESPIRATION

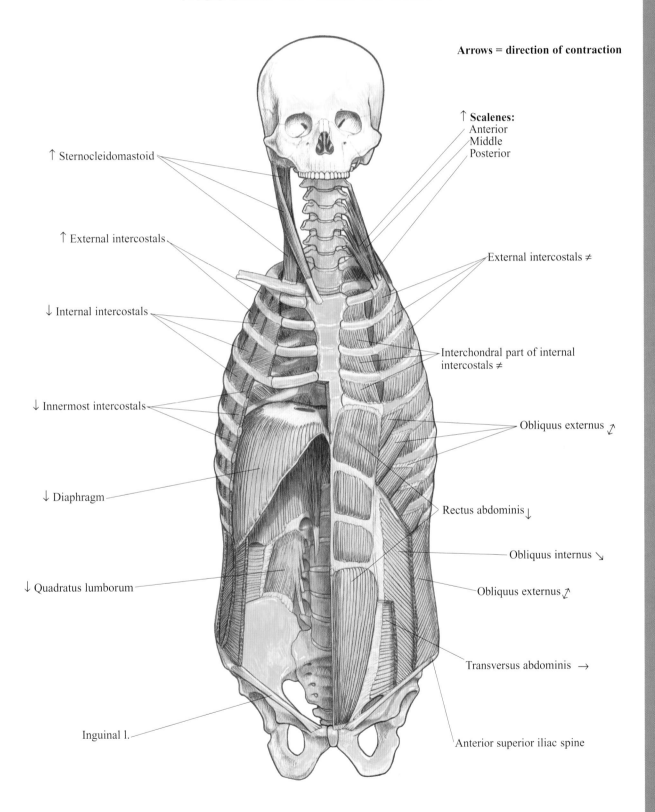

Arrows = direction of contraction

↑ Sternocleidomastoid

↑ External intercostals

↓ Internal intercostals

↓ Innermost intercostals

↓ Diaphragm

↓ Quadratus lumborum

Inguinal l.

↑ **Scalenes:**
Anterior
Middle
Posterior

External intercostals ≠

Interchondral part of internal intercostals ≠

Obliquus externus ↗

Rectus abdominis ↓

Obliquus internus ↘

Obliquus externus ↗

Transversus abdominis →

Anterior superior iliac spine

ALVEOLI CLUSTER

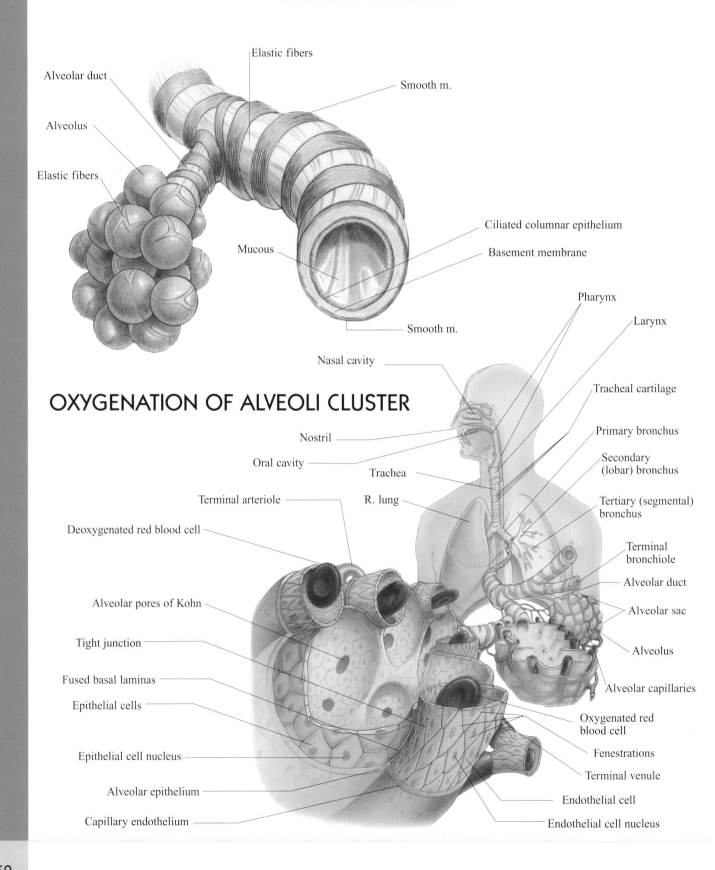

Elastic fibers

Alveolar duct

Alveolus

Elastic fibers

Smooth m.

Ciliated columnar epithelium

Basement membrane

Mucous

Smooth m.

Pharynx

Larynx

Nasal cavity

Tracheal cartilage

OXYGENATION OF ALVEOLI CLUSTER

Nostril

Oral cavity

Trachea

Primary bronchus

Secondary (lobar) bronchus

Terminal arteriole

R. lung

Tertiary (segmental) bronchus

Deoxygenated red blood cell

Terminal bronchiole

Alveolar duct

Alveolar pores of Kohn

Alveolar sac

Tight junction

Alveolus

Fused basal laminas

Epithelial cells

Alveolar capillaries

Epithelial cell nucleus

Oxygenated red blood cell

Alveolar epithelium

Fenestrations

Terminal venule

Capillary endothelium

Endothelial cell

Endothelial cell nucleus

NOTES

11

CIRCULATORY SYSTEM

CIRCULATORY SYSTEM

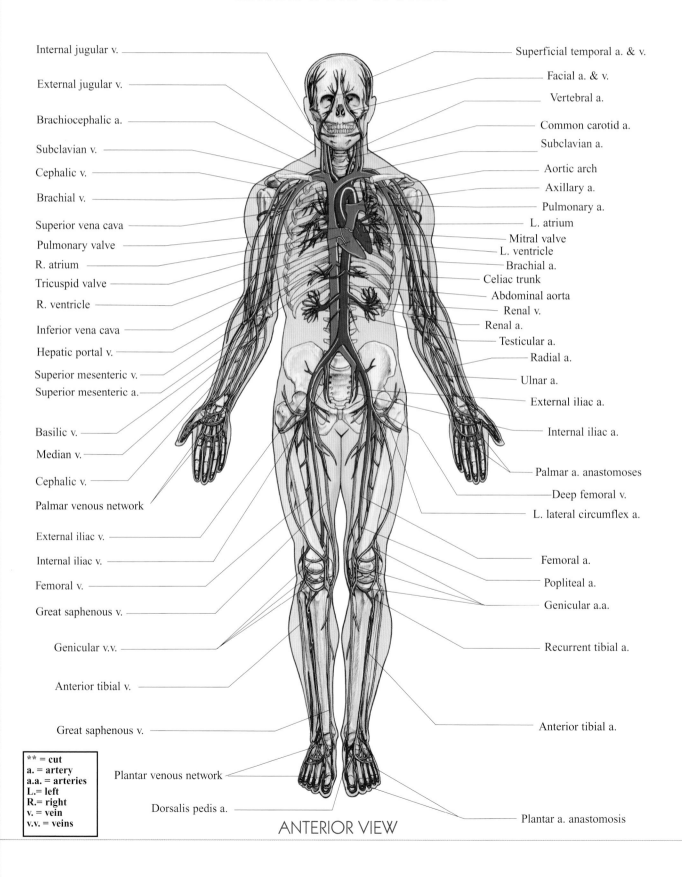

Internal jugular v.

External jugular v.

Brachiocephalic a.

Subclavian v.

Cephalic v.

Brachial v.

Superior vena cava

Pulmonary valve

R. atrium

Tricuspid valve

R. ventricle

Inferior vena cava

Hepatic portal v.

Superior mesenteric v.

Superior mesenteric a.

Basilic v.

Median v.

Cephalic v.

Palmar venous network

External iliac v.

Internal iliac v.

Femoral v.

Great saphenous v.

Genicular v.v.

Anterior tibial v.

Great saphenous v.

Plantar venous network

Dorsalis pedis a.

Superficial temporal a. & v.

Facial a. & v.

Vertebral a.

Common carotid a.

Subclavian a.

Aortic arch

Axillary a.

Pulmonary a.

L. atrium

Mitral valve

L. ventricle

Brachial a.

Celiac trunk

Abdominal aorta

Renal v.

Renal a.

Testicular a.

Radial a.

Ulnar a.

External iliac a.

Internal iliac a.

Palmar a. anastomoses

Deep femoral v.

L. lateral circumflex a.

Femoral a.

Popliteal a.

Genicular a.a.

Recurrent tibial a.

Anterior tibial a.

Plantar a. anastomosis

** = cut
a. = artery
a.a. = arteries
L.= left
R.= right
v. = vein
v.v. = veins

ANTERIOR VIEW

CIRCULATORY SYSTEM

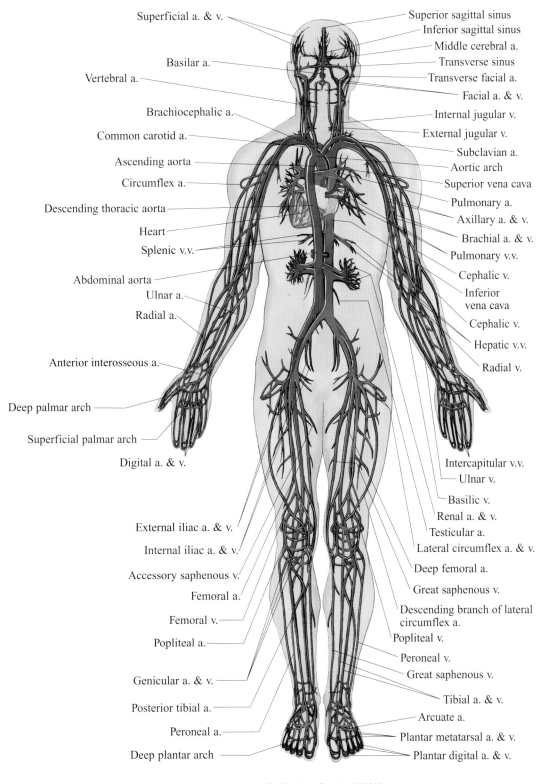

Superficial a. & v.

Basilar a.

Vertebral a.

Brachiocephalic a.

Common carotid a.

Ascending aorta

Circumflex a.

Descending thoracic aorta

Heart

Splenic v.v.

Abdominal aorta

Ulnar a.

Radial a.

Anterior interosseous a.

Deep palmar arch

Superficial palmar arch

Digital a. & v.

External iliac a. & v.

Internal iliac a. & v.

Accessory saphenous v.

Femoral a.

Femoral v.

Popliteal a.

Genicular a. & v.

Posterior tibial a.

Peroneal a.

Deep plantar arch

Superior sagittal sinus

Inferior sagittal sinus

Middle cerebral a.

Transverse sinus

Transverse facial a.

Facial a. & v.

Internal jugular v.

External jugular v.

Subclavian a.

Aortic arch

Superior vena cava

Pulmonary a.

Axillary a. & v.

Brachial a. & v.

Pulmonary v.v.

Cephalic v.

Inferior vena cava

Cephalic v.

Hepatic v.v.

Radial v.

Intercapitular v.v.

Ulnar v.

Basilic v.

Renal a. & v.

Testicular a.

Lateral circumflex a. & v.

Deep femoral a.

Great saphenous v.

Descending branch of lateral circumflex a.

Popliteal v.

Peroneal v.

Great saphenous v.

Tibial a. & v.

Arcuate a.

Plantar metatarsal a. & v.

Plantar digital a. & v.

POSTERIOR VIEW

VENOUS SYSTEM

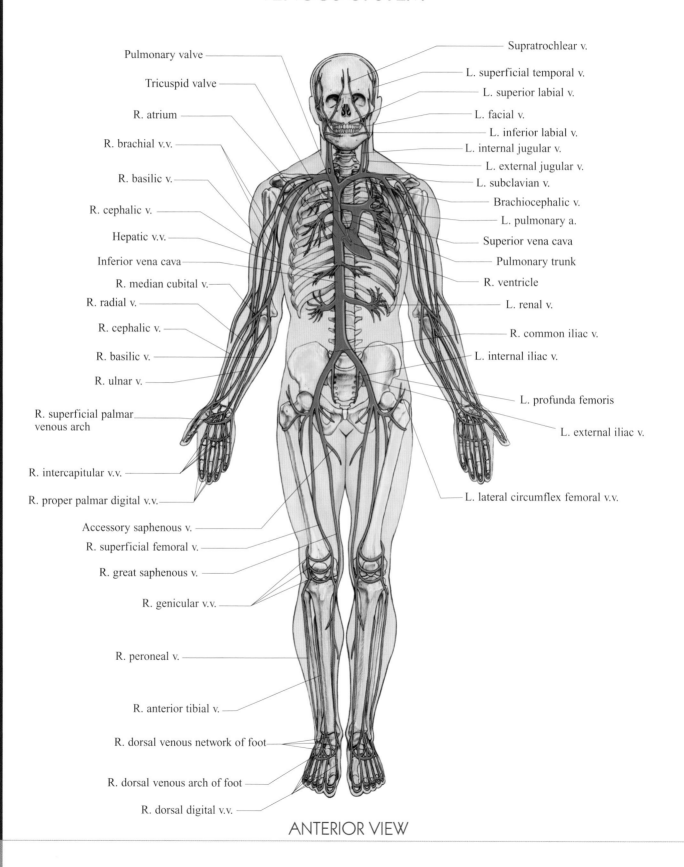

Pulmonary valve

Tricuspid valve

R. atrium

R. brachial v.v.

R. basilic v.

R. cephalic v.

Hepatic v.v.

Inferior vena cava

R. median cubital v.

R. radial v.

R. cephalic v.

R. basilic v.

R. ulnar v.

R. superficial palmar venous arch

R. intercapitular v.v.

R. proper palmar digital v.v.

Accessory saphenous v.

R. superficial femoral v.

R. great saphenous v.

R. genicular v.v.

R. peroneal v.

R. anterior tibial v.

R. dorsal venous network of foot

R. dorsal venous arch of foot

R. dorsal digital v.v.

Supratrochlear v.

L. superficial temporal v.

L. superior labial v.

L. facial v.

L. inferior labial v.

L. internal jugular v.

L. external jugular v.

L. subclavian v.

Brachiocephalic v.

L. pulmonary a.

Superior vena cava

Pulmonary trunk

R. ventricle

L. renal v.

R. common iliac v.

L. internal iliac v.

L. profunda femoris

L. external iliac v.

L. lateral circumflex femoral v.v.

ANTERIOR VIEW

ARTERIAL SYSTEM

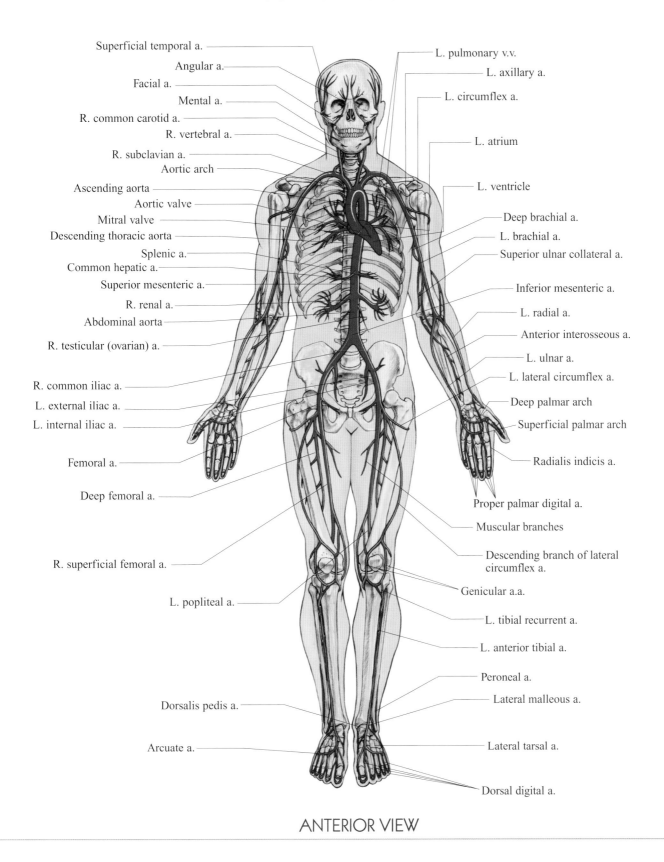

Superficial temporal a.

Angular a.

Facial a.

Mental a.

R. common carotid a.

R. vertebral a.

R. subclavian a.

Aortic arch

Ascending aorta

Aortic valve

Mitral valve

Descending thoracic aorta

Splenic a.

Common hepatic a.

Superior mesenteric a.

R. renal a.

Abdominal aorta

R. testicular (ovarian) a.

R. common iliac a.

L. external iliac a.

L. internal iliac a.

Femoral a.

Deep femoral a.

R. superficial femoral a.

L. popliteal a.

Dorsalis pedis a.

Arcuate a.

L. pulmonary v.v.

L. axillary a.

L. circumflex a.

L. atrium

L. ventricle

Deep brachial a.

L. brachial a.

Superior ulnar collateral a.

Inferior mesenteric a.

L. radial a.

Anterior interosseous a.

L. ulnar a.

L. lateral circumflex a.

Deep palmar arch

Superficial palmar arch

Radialis indicis a.

Proper palmar digital a.

Muscular branches

Descending branch of lateral circumflex a.

Genicular a.a.

L. tibial recurrent a.

L. anterior tibial a.

Peroneal a.

Lateral malleous a.

Lateral tarsal a.

Dorsal digital a.

ANTERIOR VIEW

HEAD & NECK
(SCHEMATIC)

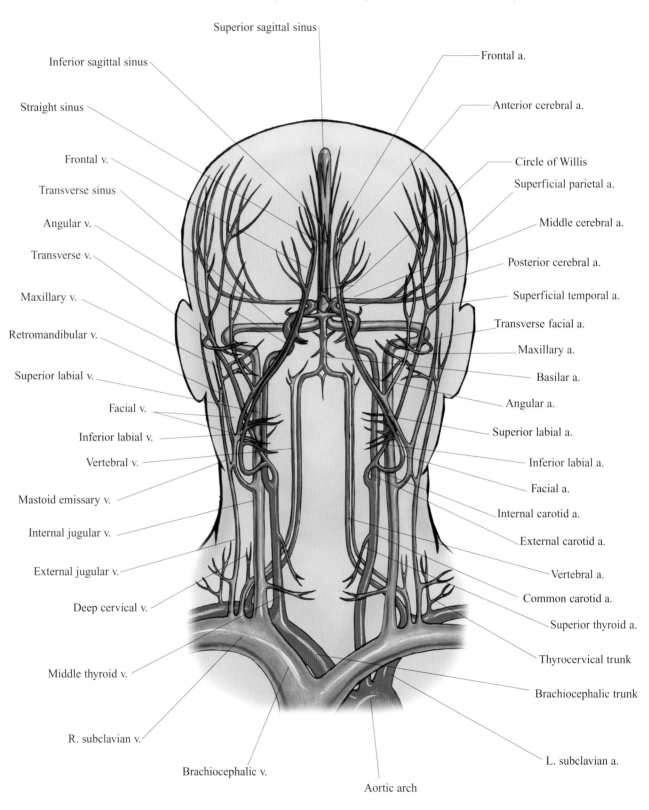

Superior sagittal sinus

Inferior sagittal sinus

Straight sinus

Frontal v.

Transverse sinus

Angular v.

Transverse v.

Maxillary v.

Retromandibular v.

Superior labial v.

Facial v.

Inferior labial v.

Vertebral v.

Mastoid emissary v.

Internal jugular v.

External jugular v.

Deep cervical v.

Middle thyroid v.

R. subclavian v.

Brachiocephalic v.

Frontal a.

Anterior cerebral a.

Circle of Willis

Superficial parietal a.

Middle cerebral a.

Posterior cerebral a.

Superficial temporal a.

Transverse facial a.

Maxillary a.

Basilar a.

Angular a.

Superior labial a.

Inferior labial a.

Facial a.

Internal carotid a.

External carotid a.

Vertebral a.

Common carotid a.

Superior thyroid a.

Thyrocervical trunk

Brachiocephalic trunk

L. subclavian a.

Aortic arch

CIRCULATORY SYSTEM

SKULL & ARTERIES

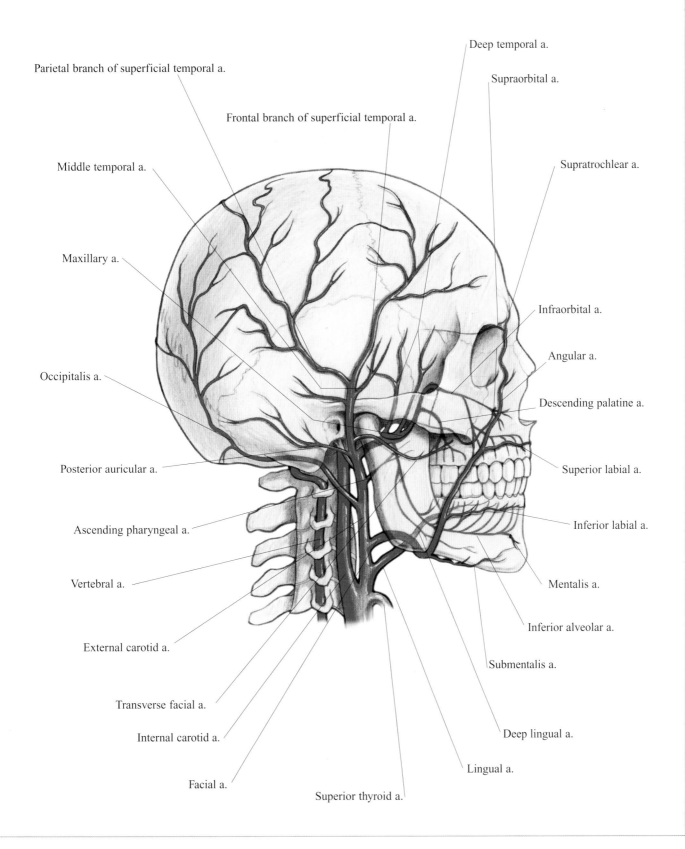

Deep temporal a.

Supraorbital a.

Parietal branch of superficial temporal a.

Supratrochlear a.

Frontal branch of superficial temporal a.

Middle temporal a.

Maxillary a.

Infraorbital a.

Angular a.

Occipitalis a.

Descending palatine a.

Posterior auricular a.

Superior labial a.

Ascending pharyngeal a.

Inferior labial a.

Vertebral a.

Mentalis a.

External carotid a.

Inferior alveolar a.

Transverse facial a.

Submentalis a.

Internal carotid a.

Deep lingual a.

Facial a.

Lingual a.

Superior thyroid a.

ARTERIES OF BRAIN & CIRCLE OF WILLIS

INFERIOR VIEW

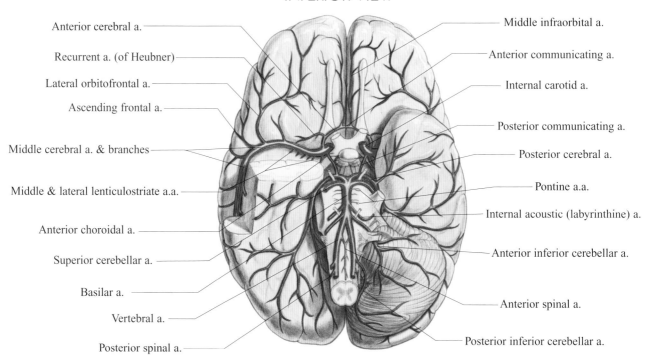

Anterior cerebral a.

Recurrent a. (of Heubner)

Lateral orbitofrontal a.

Ascending frontal a.

Middle cerebral a. & branches

Middle & lateral lenticulostriate a.a.

Anterior choroidal a.

Superior cerebellar a.

Basilar a.

Vertebral a.

Posterior spinal a.

Middle infraorbital a.

Anterior communicating a.

Internal carotid a.

Posterior communicating a.

Posterior cerebral a.

Pontine a.a.

Internal acoustic (labyrinthine) a.

Anterior inferior cerebellar a.

Anterior spinal a.

Posterior inferior cerebellar a.

CIRCLE OF WILLIS

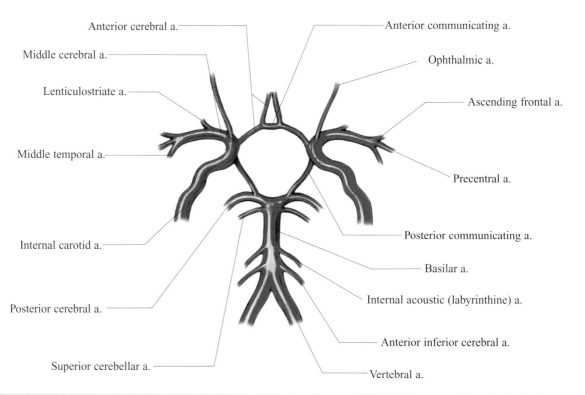

Anterior cerebral a.

Middle cerebral a.

Lenticulostriate a.

Middle temporal a.

Internal carotid a.

Posterior cerebral a.

Superior cerebellar a.

Anterior communicating a.

Ophthalmic a.

Ascending frontal a.

Precentral a.

Posterior communicating a.

Basilar a.

Internal acoustic (labyrinthine) a.

Anterior inferior cerebral a.

Vertebral a.

BRAIN & NECK

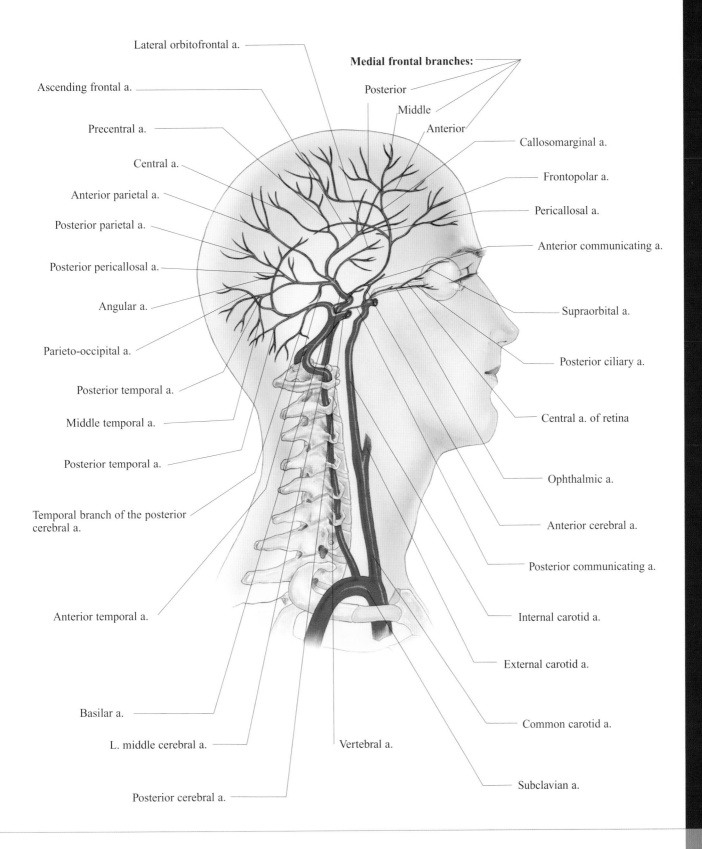

Lateral orbitofrontal a.

Ascending frontal a.

Precentral a.

Central a.

Anterior parietal a.

Posterior parietal a.

Posterior pericallosal a.

Angular a.

Parieto-occipital a.

Posterior temporal a.

Middle temporal a.

Posterior temporal a.

Temporal branch of the posterior cerebral a.

Anterior temporal a.

Basilar a.

L. middle cerebral a.

Posterior cerebral a.

Medial frontal branches:

Posterior

Middle

Anterior

Callosomarginal a.

Frontopolar a.

Pericallosal a.

Anterior communicating a.

Supraorbital a.

Posterior ciliary a.

Central a. of retina

Ophthalmic a.

Anterior cerebral a.

Posterior communicating a.

Internal carotid a.

External carotid a.

Common carotid a.

Vertebral a.

Subclavian a.

BLOOD CIRCUITS

Veins (Blood flows *toward* heart)   **Arteries** (Blood flows *away from* heart)

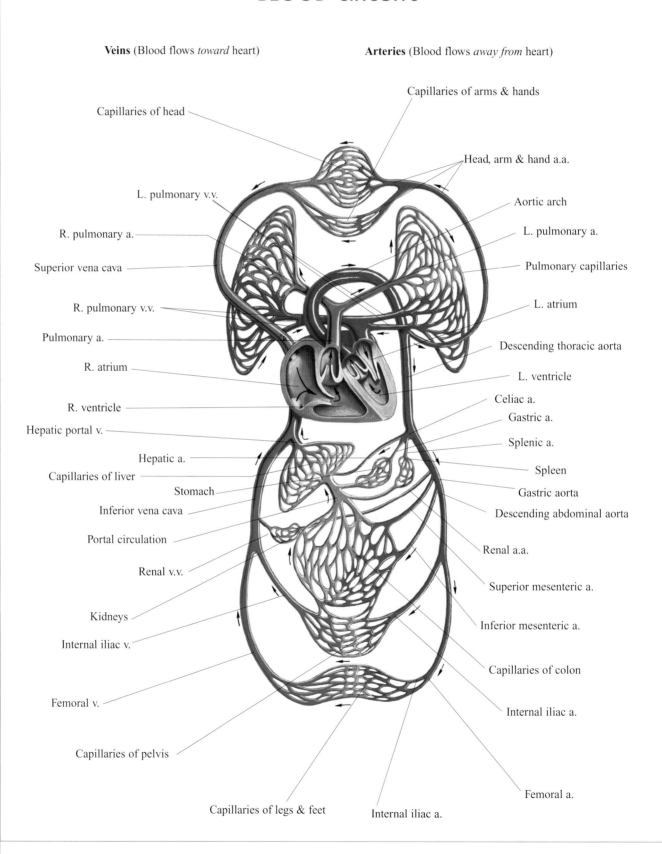

Capillaries of head

Capillaries of arms & hands

Head, arm & hand a.a.

L. pulmonary v.v.

Aortic arch

R. pulmonary a.

L. pulmonary a.

Superior vena cava

Pulmonary capillaries

R. pulmonary v.v.

L. atrium

Pulmonary a.

Descending thoracic aorta

R. atrium

L. ventricle

Celiac a.

R. ventricle

Gastric a.

Hepatic portal v.

Splenic a.

Hepatic a.

Spleen

Capillaries of liver

Gastric aorta

Stomach

Descending abdominal aorta

Inferior vena cava

Portal circulation

Renal a.a.

Renal v.v.

Superior mesenteric a.

Kidneys

Inferior mesenteric a.

Internal iliac v.

Capillaries of colon

Femoral v.

Internal iliac a.

Capillaries of pelvis

Femoral a.

Capillaries of legs & feet

Internal iliac a.

HEPATIC PORTAL VEINS

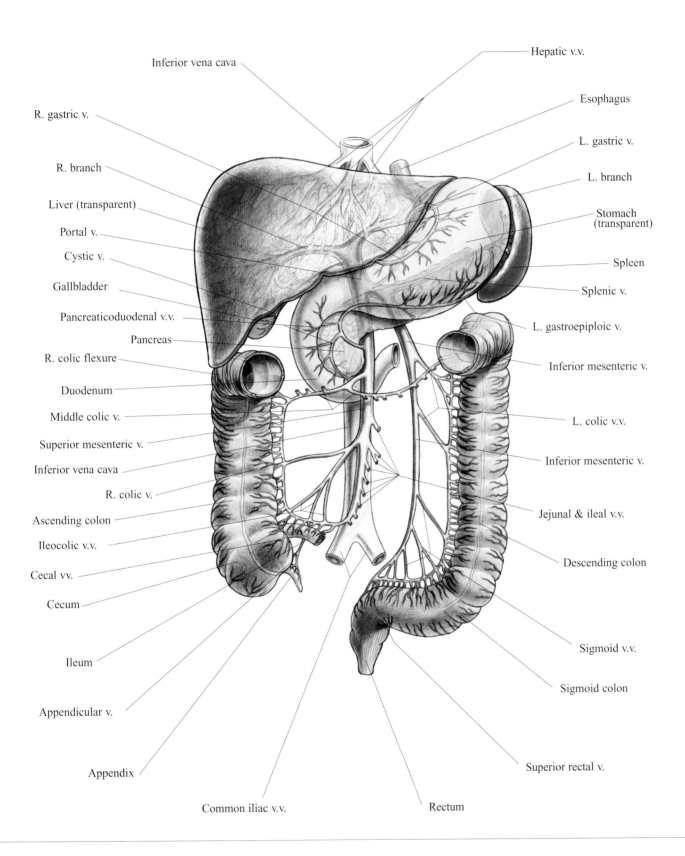

Inferior vena cava

Hepatic v.v.

Esophagus

R. gastric v.

L. gastric v.

R. branch

L. branch

Liver (transparent)

Stomach (transparent)

Portal v.

Cystic v.

Spleen

Gallbladder

Splenic v.

Pancreaticoduodenal v.v.

L. gastroepiploic v.

Pancreas

Inferior mesenteric v.

R. colic flexure

Duodenum

L. colic v.v.

Middle colic v.

Superior mesenteric v.

Inferior mesenteric v.

Inferior vena cava

R. colic v.

Jejunal & ileal v.v.

Ascending colon

Ileocolic v.v.

Descending colon

Cecal vv.

Cecum

Sigmoid v.v.

Ileum

Sigmoid colon

Appendicular v.

Superior rectal v.

Appendix

Common iliac v.v.

Rectum

BLOOD VESSELS

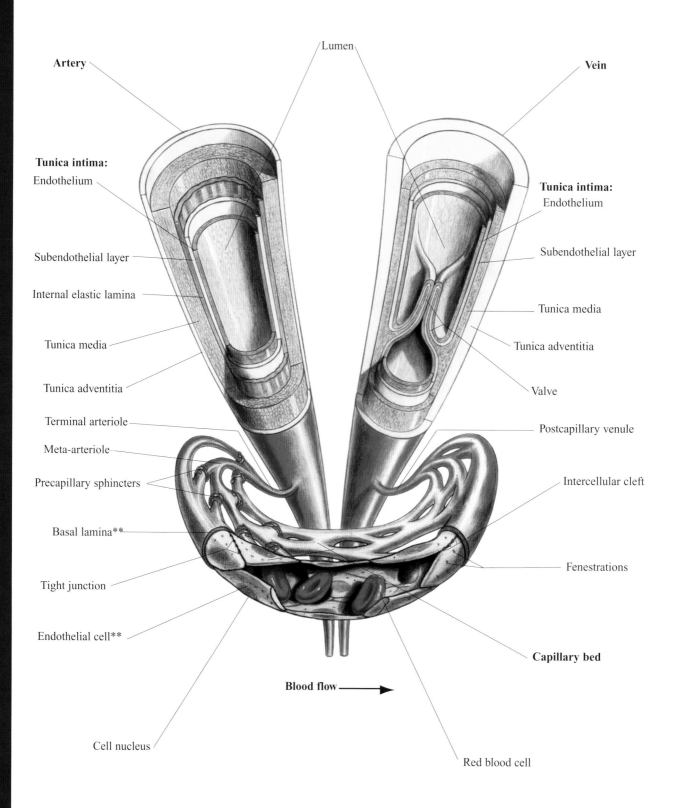

Artery

Lumen

Vein

Tunica intima:
Endothelium

Subendothelial layer

Internal elastic lamina

Tunica media

Tunica adventitia

Terminal arteriole

Meta-arteriole

Precapillary sphincters

Basal lamina**

Tight junction

Endothelial cell**

Cell nucleus

Tunica intima:
Endothelium

Subendothelial layer

Tunica media

Tunica adventitia

Valve

Postcapillary venule

Intercellular cleft

Fenestrations

Capillary bed

Red blood cell

Blood flow ⟶

NOTES

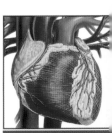

12

THE HEART

HEART

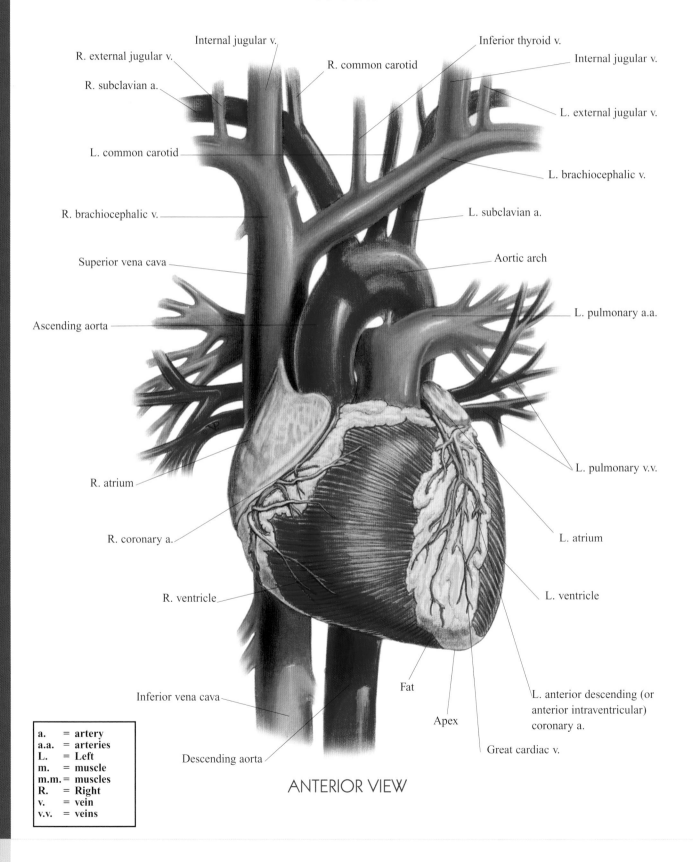

Internal jugular v.

R. external jugular v.

R. subclavian a.

R. common carotid

Inferior thyroid v.

Internal jugular v.

L. external jugular v.

L. common carotid

R. brachiocephalic v.

Superior vena cava

Ascending aorta

R. atrium

R. coronary a.

R. ventricle

Inferior vena cava

Descending aorta

L. brachiocephalic v.

L. subclavian a.

Aortic arch

L. pulmonary a.a.

L. pulmonary v.v.

L. atrium

L. ventricle

Fat

Apex

Great cardiac v.

L. anterior descending (or anterior intraventricular) coronary a.

a.	=	artery
a.a.	=	arteries
L.	=	Left
m.	=	muscle
m.m.	=	muscles
R.	=	Right
v.	=	vein
v.v.	=	veins

ANTERIOR VIEW

HEART

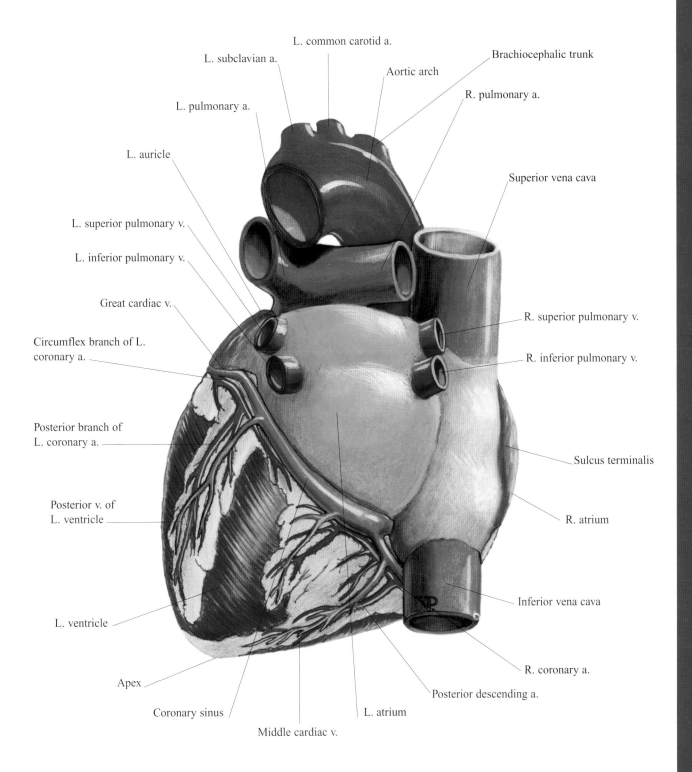

L. common carotid a.

L. subclavian a.

Aortic arch

Brachiocephalic trunk

R. pulmonary a.

L. pulmonary a.

L. auricle

Superior vena cava

L. superior pulmonary v.

L. inferior pulmonary v.

Great cardiac v.

R. superior pulmonary v.

Circumflex branch of L. coronary a.

R. inferior pulmonary v.

Posterior branch of L. coronary a.

Sulcus terminalis

Posterior v. of L. ventricle

R. atrium

L. ventricle

Inferior vena cava

Apex

R. coronary a.

Coronary sinus

Posterior descending a.

Middle cardiac v.

L. atrium

POSTERIOR VIEW

CORONARY ARTERIES & CARDIAC VEINS

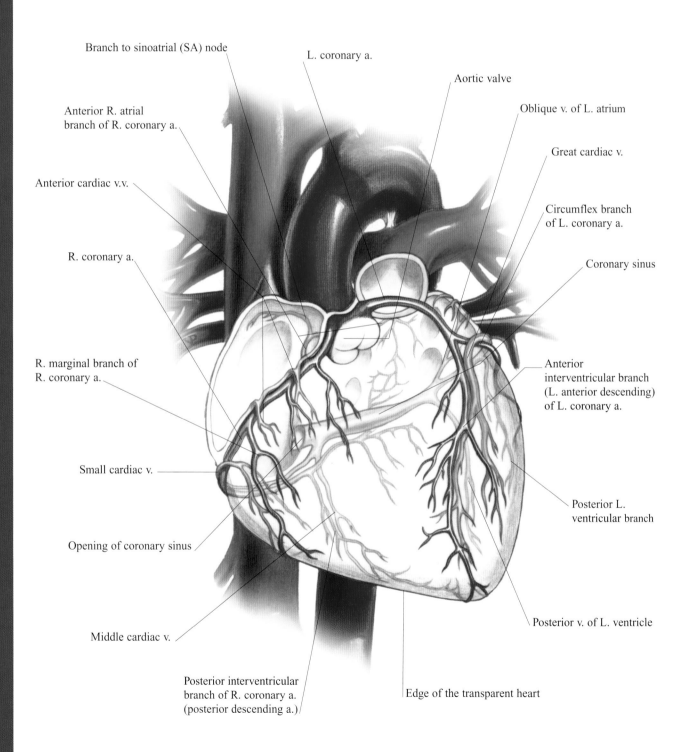

Branch to sinoatrial (SA) node

L. coronary a.

Aortic valve

Anterior R. atrial
branch of R. coronary a.

Oblique v. of L. atrium

Great cardiac v.

Anterior cardiac v.v.

Circumflex branch
of L. coronary a.

R. coronary a.

Coronary sinus

R. marginal branch of
R. coronary a.

Anterior
interventricular branch
(L. anterior descending)
of L. coronary a.

Small cardiac v.

Opening of coronary sinus

Posterior L.
ventricular branch

Posterior v. of L. ventricle

Middle cardiac v.

Posterior interventricular
branch of R. coronary a.
(posterior descending a.)

Edge of the transparent heart

HEART

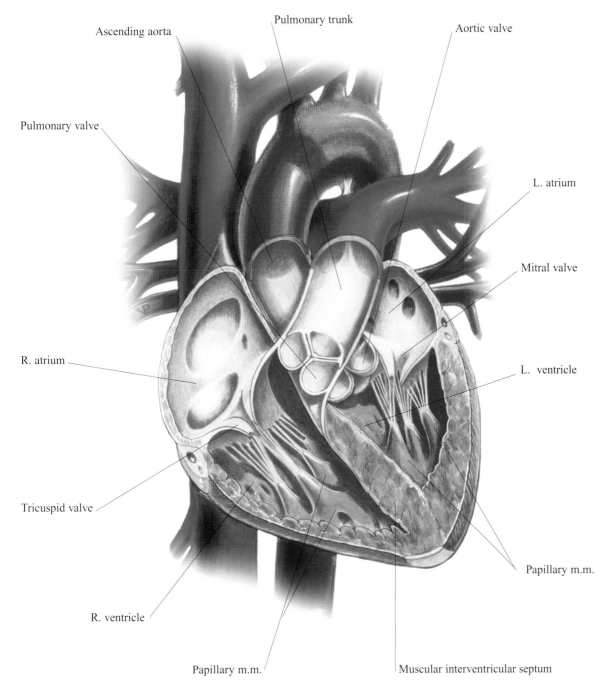

Ascending aorta

Pulmonary trunk

Aortic valve

Pulmonary valve

L. atrium

Mitral valve

R. atrium

L. ventricle

Tricuspid valve

Papillary m.m.

R. ventricle

Papillary m.m.

Muscular interventricular septum

INTERIOR VIEW

CIRCULATION

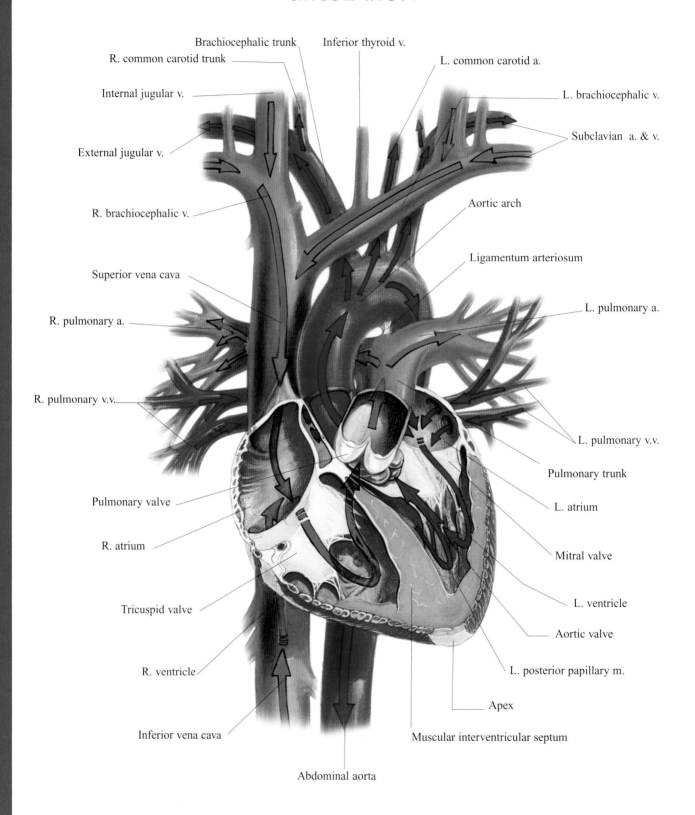

Brachiocephalic trunk

R. common carotid trunk

Internal jugular v.

External jugular v.

R. brachiocephalic v.

Superior vena cava

R. pulmonary a.

R. pulmonary v.v.

Pulmonary valve

R. atrium

Tricuspid valve

R. ventricle

Inferior vena cava

Abdominal aorta

Inferior thyroid v.

L. common carotid a.

L. brachiocephalic v.

Subclavian a. & v.

Aortic arch

Ligamentum arteriosum

L. pulmonary a.

L. pulmonary v.v.

Pulmonary trunk

L. atrium

Mitral valve

L. ventricle

Aortic valve

L. posterior papillary m.

Apex

Muscular interventricular septum

NERVES & ARTERIES

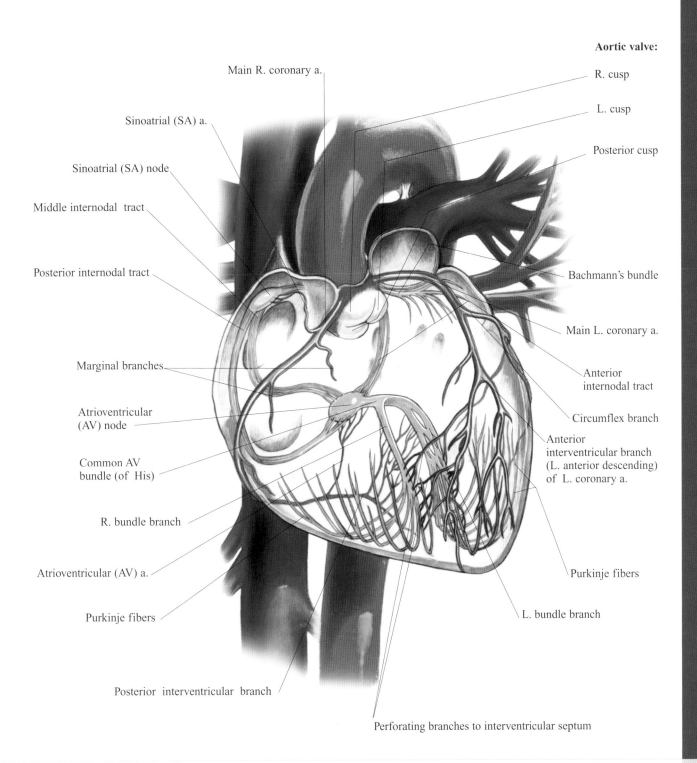

Main R. coronary a.

Sinoatrial (SA) a.

Sinoatrial (SA) node

Middle internodal tract

Posterior internodal tract

Marginal branches

Atrioventricular (AV) node

Common AV bundle (of His)

R. bundle branch

Atrioventricular (AV) a.

Purkinje fibers

Posterior interventricular branch

Aortic valve:

R. cusp

L. cusp

Posterior cusp

Bachmann's bundle

Main L. coronary a.

Anterior internodal tract

Circumflex branch

Anterior interventricular branch (L. anterior descending) of L. coronary a.

Purkinje fibers

L. bundle branch

Perforating branches to interventricular septum

HEART IN DIASTOLE

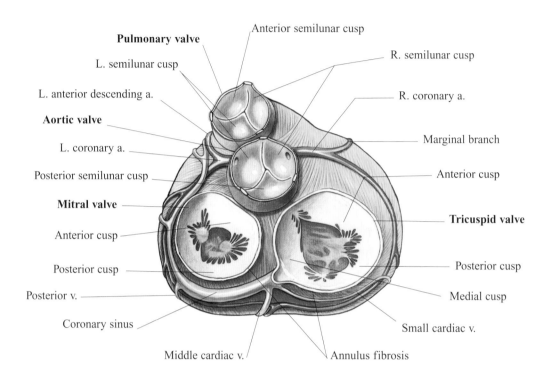

Pulmonary valve

L. semilunar cusp

L. anterior descending a.

Aortic valve

L. coronary a.

Posterior semilunar cusp

Mitral valve

Anterior cusp

Posterior cusp

Posterior v.

Coronary sinus

Middle cardiac v.

Anterior semilunar cusp

R. semilunar cusp

R. coronary a.

Marginal branch

Anterior cusp

Tricuspid valve

Posterior cusp

Medial cusp

Small cardiac v.

Annulus fibrosis

HEART IN SYSTOLE

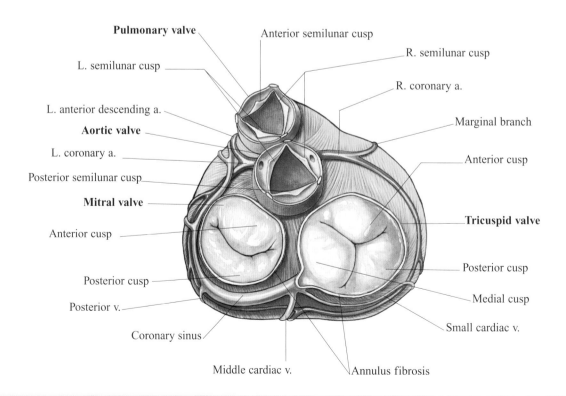

Pulmonary valve

L. semilunar cusp

L. anterior descending a.

Aortic valve

L. coronary a.

Posterior semilunar cusp

Mitral valve

Anterior cusp

Posterior cusp

Posterior v.

Coronary sinus

Middle cardiac v.

Anterior semilunar cusp

R. semilunar cusp

R. coronary a.

Marginal branch

Anterior cusp

Tricuspid valve

Posterior cusp

Medial cusp

Small cardiac v.

Annulus fibrosis

BEGINNING OF DIASTOLE

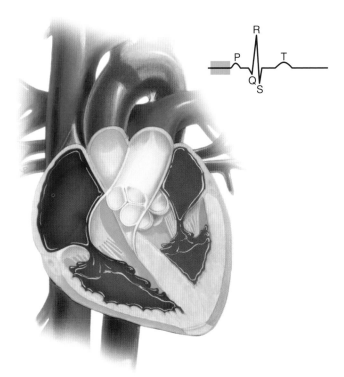

END OF DIASTOLE

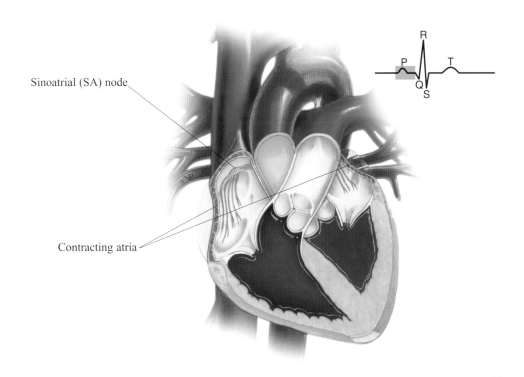

Sinoatrial (SA) node

Contracting atria

BEGINNING OF SYSTOLE

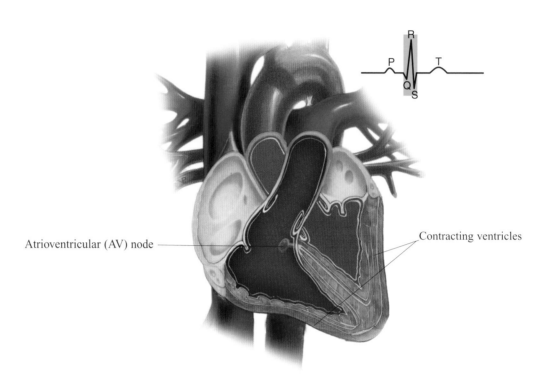

Atrioventricular (AV) node

Contracting ventricles

END OF SYSTOLE

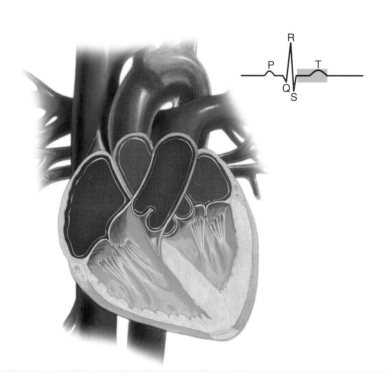

NOTES

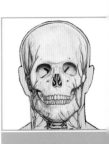

13

LYMPHATIC SYSTEM

LYMPHATIC SYSTEM

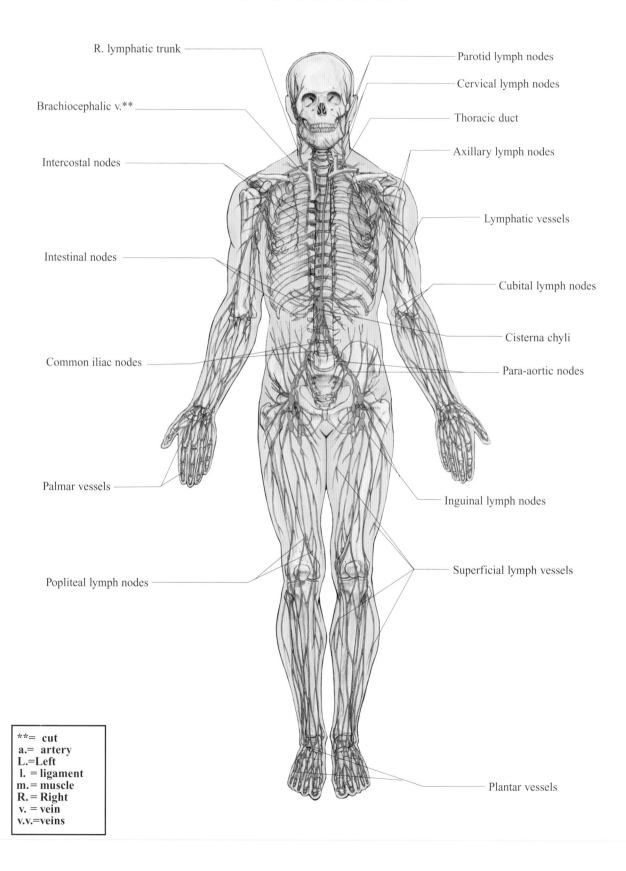

R. lymphatic trunk

Brachiocephalic v.**

Intercostal nodes

Intestinal nodes

Common iliac nodes

Palmar vessels

Popliteal lymph nodes

Parotid lymph nodes

Cervical lymph nodes

Thoracic duct

Axillary lymph nodes

Lymphatic vessels

Cubital lymph nodes

Cisterna chyli

Para-aortic nodes

Inguinal lymph nodes

Superficial lymph vessels

Plantar vessels

**= cut
a.= artery
L.=Left
l. = ligament
m.= muscle
R. = Right
v. = vein
v.v.=veins

HEAD & NECK

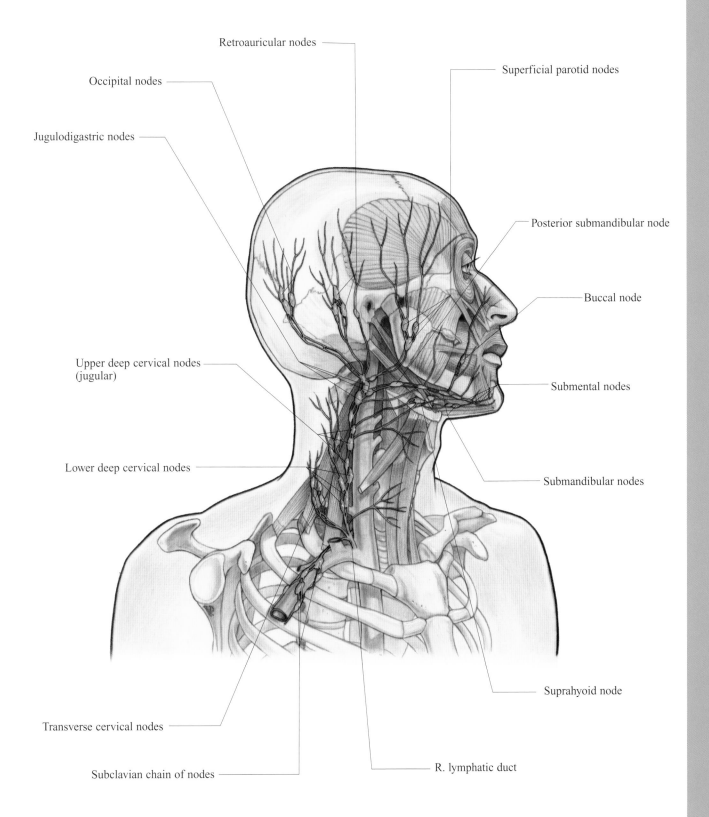

Retroauricular nodes

Occipital nodes

Jugulodigastric nodes

Superficial parotid nodes

Posterior submandibular node

Buccal node

Upper deep cervical nodes
(jugular)

Lower deep cervical nodes

Submental nodes

Submandibular nodes

Suprahyoid node

Transverse cervical nodes

Subclavian chain of nodes

R. lymphatic duct

ARM AXILLA & THORAX

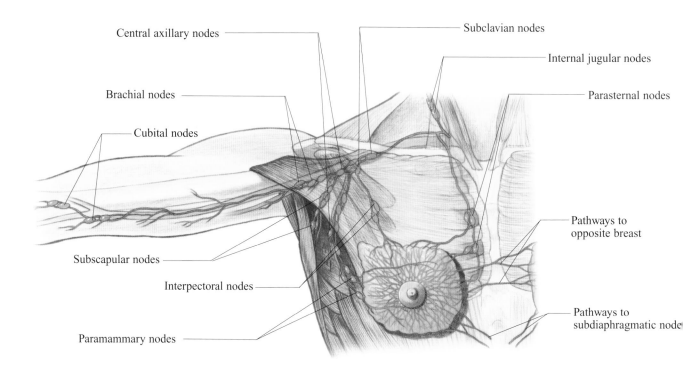

Central axillary nodes

Subclavian nodes

Internal jugular nodes

Brachial nodes

Parasternal nodes

Cubital nodes

Pathways to
opposite breast

Subscapular nodes

Interpectoral nodes

Pathways to
subdiaphragmatic node

Paramammary nodes

HEART & LUNGS

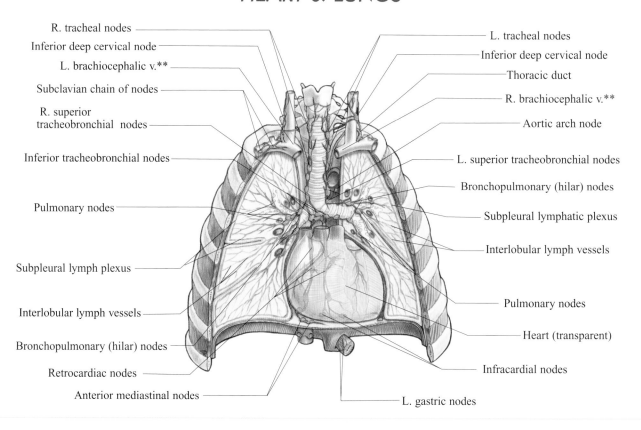

R. tracheal nodes

L. tracheal nodes

Inferior deep cervical node

Inferior deep cervical node

L. brachiocephalic v.**

Thoracic duct

Subclavian chain of nodes

R. brachiocephalic v.**

R. superior
tracheobronchial nodes

Aortic arch node

Inferior tracheobronchial nodes

L. superior tracheobronchial nodes

Bronchopulmonary (hilar) nodes

Pulmonary nodes

Subpleural lymphatic plexus

Interlobular lymph vessels

Subpleural lymph plexus

Interlobular lymph vessels

Pulmonary nodes

Bronchopulmonary (hilar) nodes

Heart (transparent)

Retrocardiac nodes

Infracardial nodes

Anterior mediastinal nodes

L. gastric nodes

THORACIC DUCT

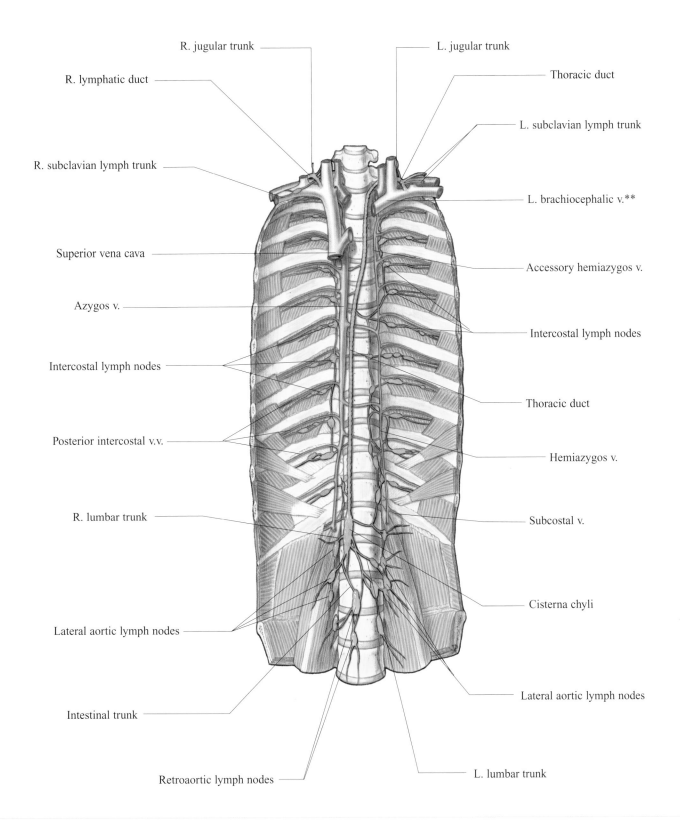

R. jugular trunk

L. jugular trunk

R. lymphatic duct

Thoracic duct

L. subclavian lymph trunk

R. subclavian lymph trunk

L. brachiocephalic v.**

Superior vena cava

Accessory hemiazygos v.

Azygos v.

Intercostal lymph nodes

Intercostal lymph nodes

Thoracic duct

Posterior intercostal v.v.

Hemiazygos v.

R. lumbar trunk

Subcostal v.

Cisterna chyli

Lateral aortic lymph nodes

Lateral aortic lymph nodes

Intestinal trunk

Retroaortic lymph nodes

L. lumbar trunk

DEEP ABDOMINAL & INGUINAL NODES

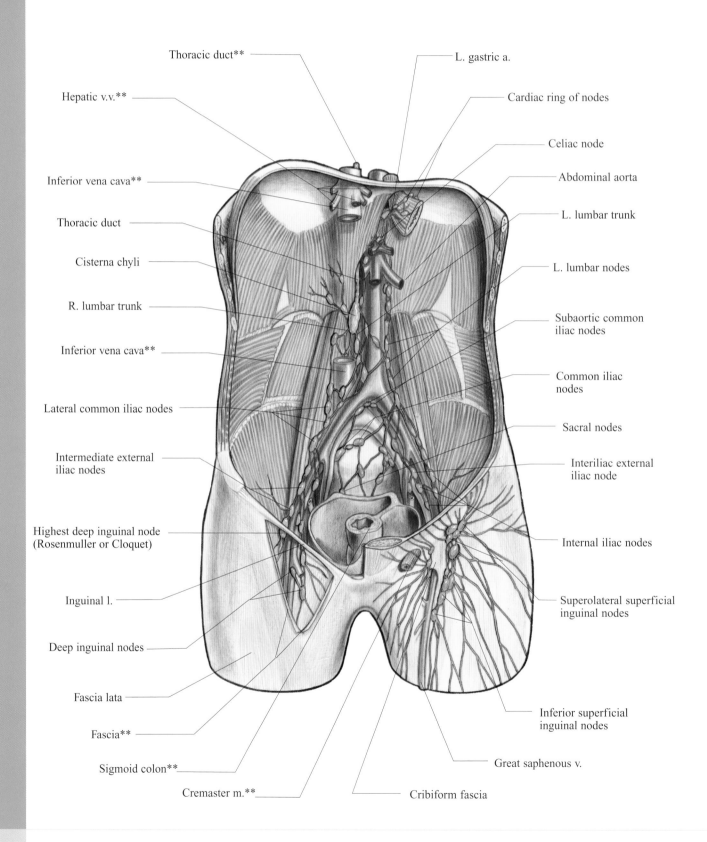

Thoracic duct**

Hepatic v.v.**

Inferior vena cava**

Thoracic duct

Cisterna chyli

R. lumbar trunk

Inferior vena cava**

Lateral common iliac nodes

Intermediate external
iliac nodes

Highest deep inguinal node
(Rosenmuller or Cloquet)

Inguinal l.

Deep inguinal nodes

Fascia lata

Fascia**

Sigmoid colon**

Cremaster m.**

L. gastric a.

Cardiac ring of nodes

Celiac node

Abdominal aorta

L. lumbar trunk

L. lumbar nodes

Subaortic common
iliac nodes

Common iliac
nodes

Sacral nodes

Interiliac external
iliac node

Internal iliac nodes

Superolateral superficial
inguinal nodes

Inferior superficial
inguinal nodes

Great saphenous v.

Cribiform fascia

STOMACH & PANCREAS

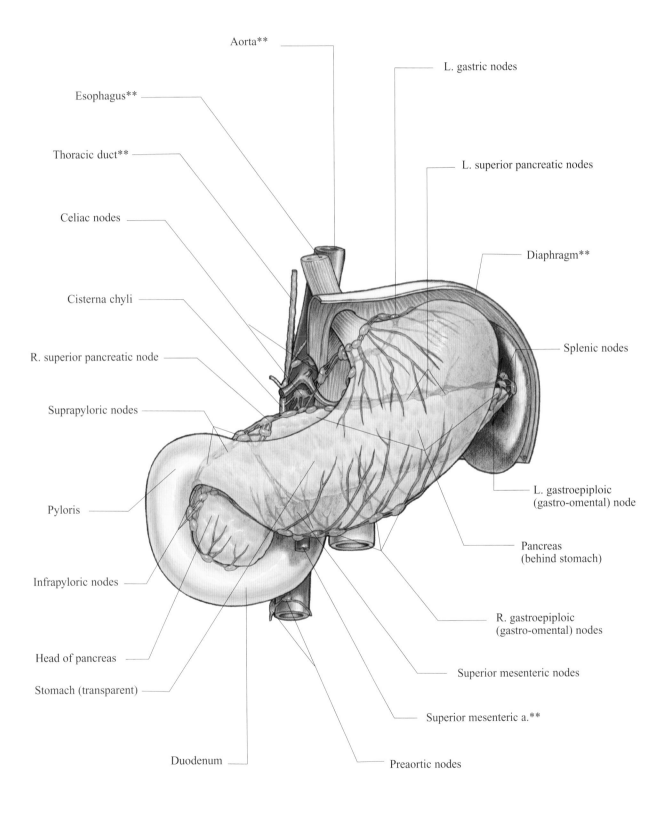

Aorta**

L. gastric nodes

Esophagus**

Thoracic duct**

L. superior pancreatic nodes

Celiac nodes

Cisterna chyli

Diaphragm**

R. superior pancreatic node

Splenic nodes

Suprapyloric nodes

Pyloris

L. gastroepiploic
(gastro-omental) node

Infrapyloric nodes

Pancreas
(behind stomach)

Head of pancreas

R. gastroepiploic
(gastro-omental) nodes

Stomach (transparent)

Superior mesenteric nodes

Duodenum

Superior mesenteric a.**

Preaortic nodes

LARGE INTESTINE

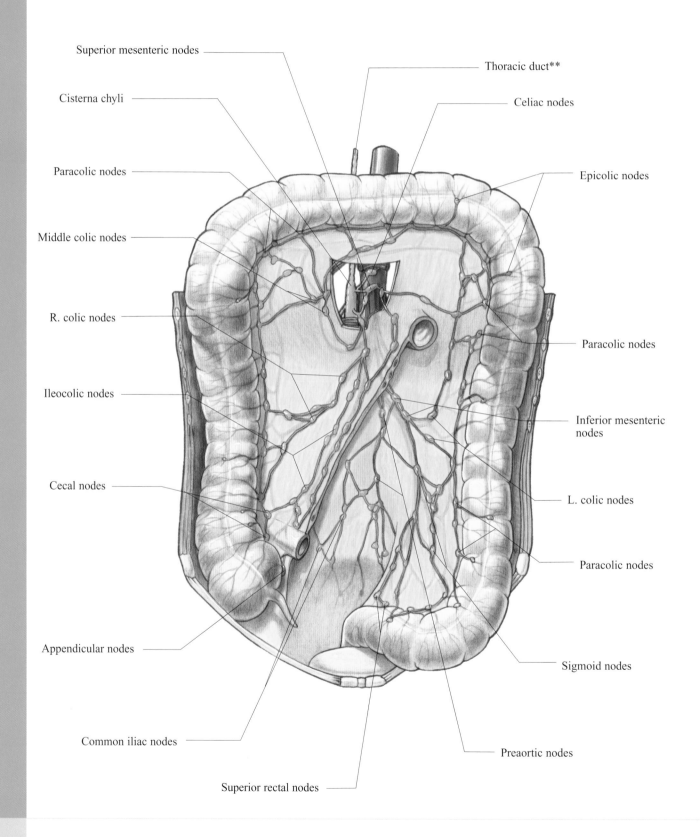

Superior mesenteric nodes

Cisterna chyli

Paracolic nodes

Middle colic nodes

R. colic nodes

Ileocolic nodes

Cecal nodes

Appendicular nodes

Common iliac nodes

Superior rectal nodes

Thoracic duct**

Celiac nodes

Epicolic nodes

Paracolic nodes

Inferior mesenteric nodes

L. colic nodes

Paracolic nodes

Sigmoid nodes

Preaortic nodes

NODES & VESSELS

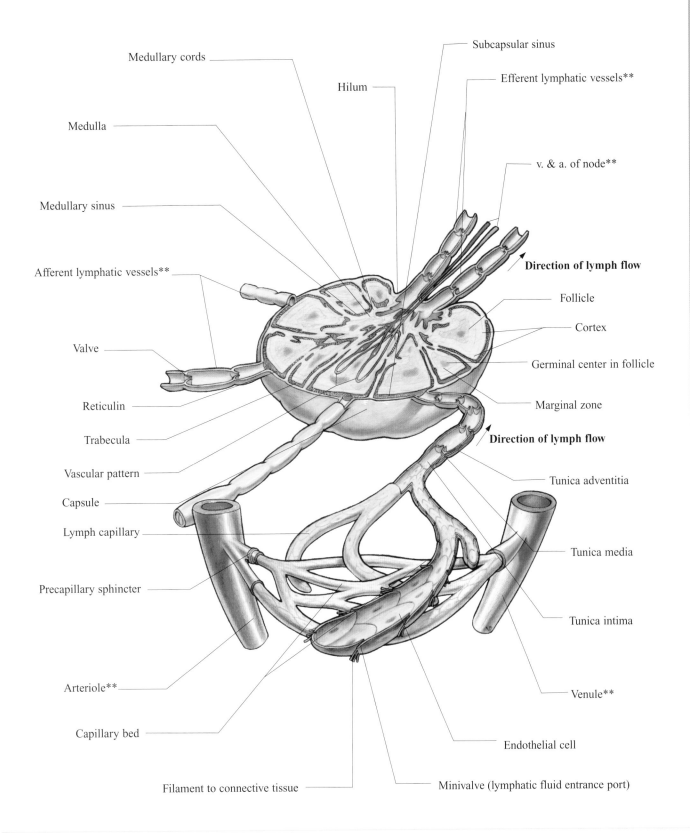

Medullary cords

Medulla

Medullary sinus

Afferent lymphatic vessels**

Valve

Reticulin

Trabecula

Vascular pattern

Capsule

Lymph capillary

Precapillary sphincter

Arteriole**

Capillary bed

Filament to connective tissue

Hilum

Subcapsular sinus

Efferent lymphatic vessels**

v. & a. of node**

Direction of lymph flow

Follicle

Cortex

Germinal center in follicle

Marginal zone

Direction of lymph flow

Tunica adventitia

Tunica media

Tunica intima

Venule**

Endothelial cell

Minivalve (lymphatic fluid entrance port)

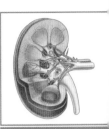

14

UROGENITAL SYSTEM

UROGENITAL SYSTEM

MALE UROGENITAL SYSTEM

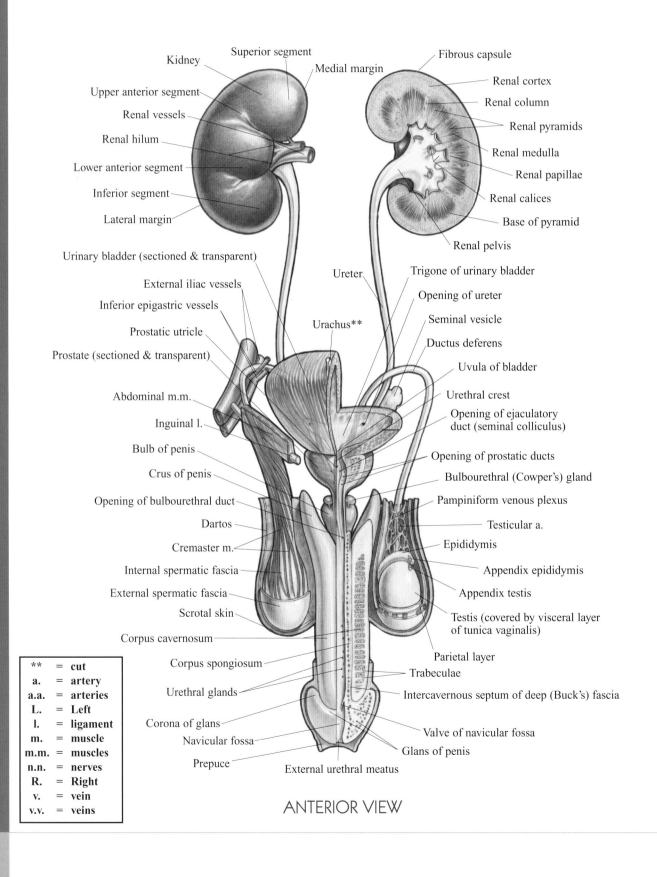

Kidney

Superior segment

Medial margin

Upper anterior segment

Renal vessels

Renal hilum

Lower anterior segment

Inferior segment

Lateral margin

Fibrous capsule

Renal cortex

Renal column

Renal pyramids

Renal medulla

Renal papillae

Renal calices

Base of pyramid

Renal pelvis

Urinary bladder (sectioned & transparent)

External iliac vessels

Inferior epigastric vessels

Prostatic utricle

Prostate (sectioned & transparent)

Abdominal m.m.

Inguinal l.

Bulb of penis

Crus of penis

Opening of bulbourethral duct

Dartos

Cremaster m.

Internal spermatic fascia

External spermatic fascia

Scrotal skin

Corpus cavernosum

Corpus spongiosum

Urethral glands

Corona of glans

Navicular fossa

Prepuce

Ureter

Urachus**

Trigone of urinary bladder

Opening of ureter

Seminal vesicle

Ductus deferens

Uvula of bladder

Urethral crest

Opening of ejaculatory duct (seminal colliculus)

Opening of prostatic ducts

Bulbourethral (Cowper's) gland

Pampiniform venous plexus

Testicular a.

Epididymis

Appendix epididymis

Appendix testis

Testis (covered by visceral layer of tunica vaginalis)

Parietal layer

Trabeculae

Intercavernous septum of deep (Buck's) fascia

Valve of navicular fossa

Glans of penis

External urethral meatus

**	=	cut
a.	=	artery
a.a.	=	arteries
L.	=	Left
l.	=	ligament
m.	=	muscle
m.m.	=	muscles
n.n.	=	nerves
R.	=	Right
v.	=	vein
v.v.	=	veins

ANTERIOR VIEW

MALE URINARY SYSTEM

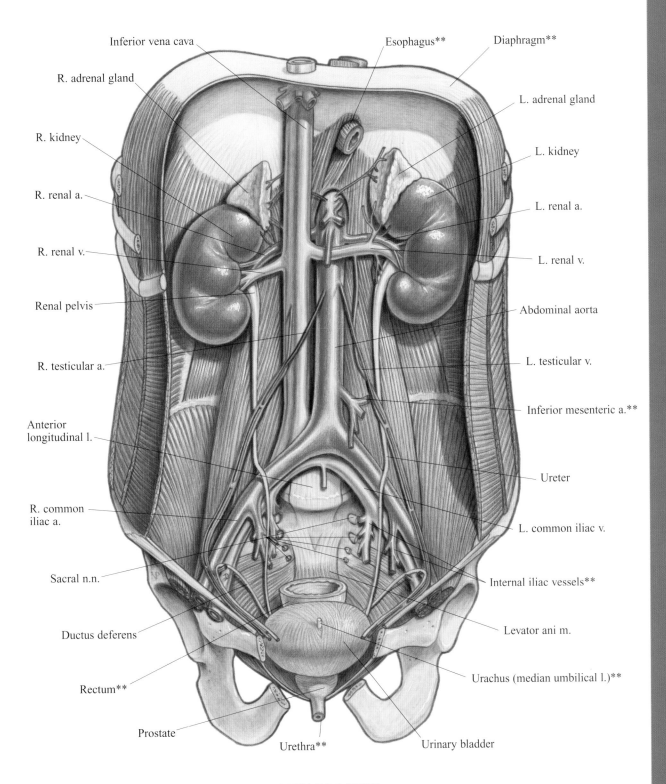

Inferior vena cava

Esophagus**

Diaphragm**

R. adrenal gland

L. adrenal gland

R. kidney

L. kidney

R. renal a.

L. renal a.

R. renal v.

L. renal v.

Renal pelvis

Abdominal aorta

R. testicular a.

L. testicular v.

Inferior mesenteric a.**

Anterior
longitudinal l.

Ureter

R. common
iliac a.

L. common iliac v.

Sacral n.n.

Internal iliac vessels**

Ductus deferens

Levator ani m.

Urachus (median umbilical l.)**

Rectum**

Prostate

Urethra**

Urinary bladder

ANTERIOR VIEW

MALE UROGENITAL SYSTEM

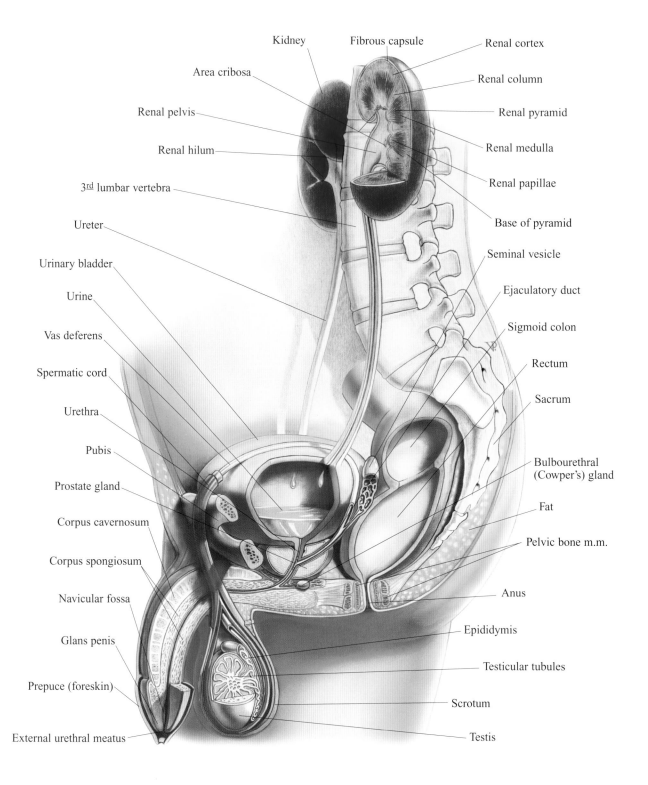

Kidney

Fibrous capsule

Renal cortex

Area cribosa

Renal column

Renal pelvis

Renal pyramid

Renal hilum

Renal medulla

3rd lumbar vertebra

Renal papillae

Base of pyramid

Ureter

Seminal vesicle

Urinary bladder

Ejaculatory duct

Urine

Sigmoid colon

Vas deferens

Rectum

Spermatic cord

Sacrum

Urethra

Pubis

Bulbourethral
(Cowper's) gland

Prostate gland

Fat

Corpus cavernosum

Pelvic bone m.m.

Corpus spongiosum

Navicular fossa

Anus

Glans penis

Epididymis

Testicular tubules

Prepuce (foreskin)

Scrotum

External urethral meatus

Testis

LATERAL VIEW

UROGENITAL SYSTEM

FEMALE UROGENITAL SYSTEM

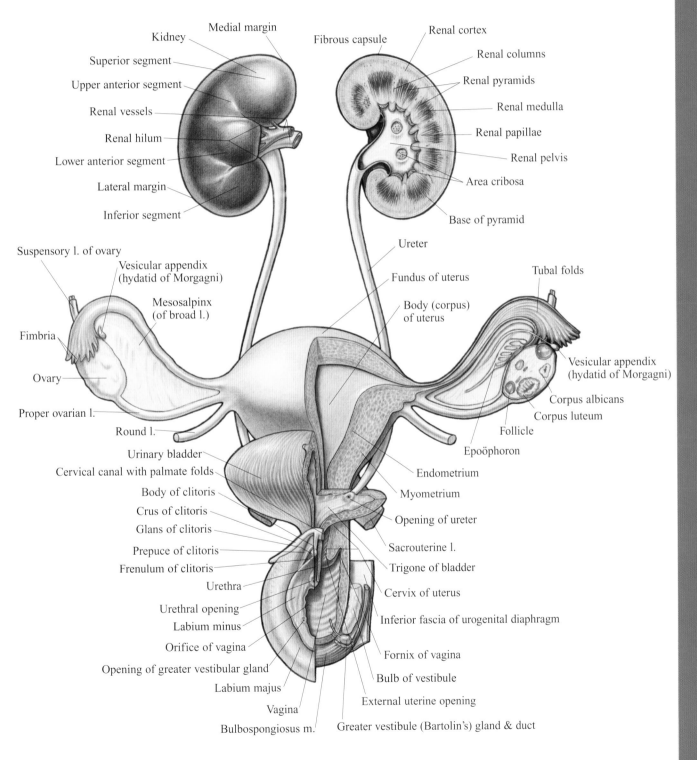

Medial margin
Kidney
Superior segment
Upper anterior segment
Renal vessels
Renal hilum
Lower anterior segment
Lateral margin
Inferior segment

Fibrous capsule
Renal cortex
Renal columns
Renal pyramids
Renal medulla
Renal papillae
Renal pelvis
Area cribosa
Base of pyramid

Suspensory l. of ovary
Vesicular appendix
(hydatid of Morgagni)
Mesosalpinx
(of broad l.)
Fimbria
Ovary
Proper ovarian l.
Round l.

Ureter
Fundus of uterus
Body (corpus)
of uterus

Tubal folds

Vesicular appendix
(hydatid of Morgagni)
Corpus albicans
Corpus luteum
Follicle
Epoöphoron

Urinary bladder
Cervical canal with palmate folds
Body of clitoris
Crus of clitoris
Glans of clitoris
Prepuce of clitoris
Frenulum of clitoris
Urethra
Urethral opening
Labium minus
Orifice of vagina
Opening of greater vestibular gland
Labium majus
Vagina
Bulbospongiosus m.

Endometrium
Myometrium
Opening of ureter
Sacrouterine l.
Trigone of bladder
Cervix of uterus
Inferior fascia of urogenital diaphragm
Fornix of vagina
Bulb of vestibule
External uterine opening
Greater vestibule (Bartolin's) gland & duct

ANTERIOR VIEW

195

FEMALE UROGENITAL SYSTEM

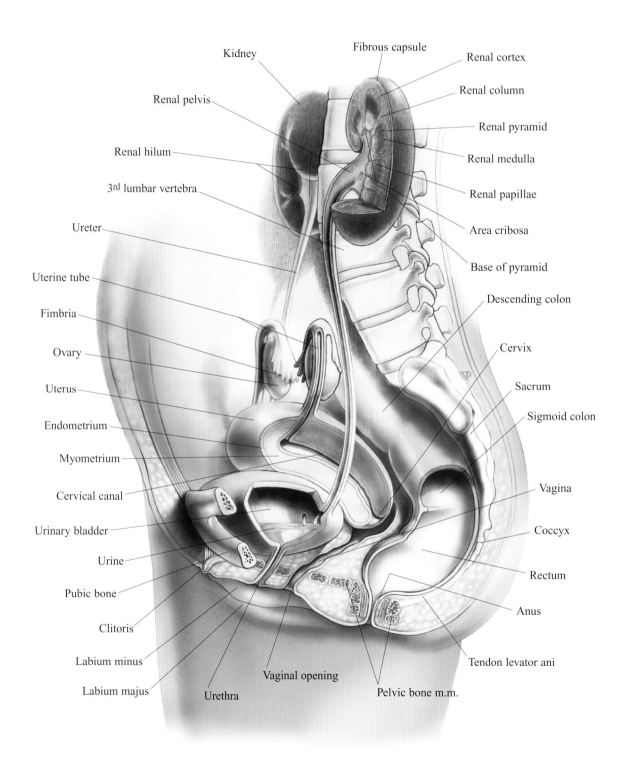

Kidney

Fibrous capsule

Renal cortex

Renal pelvis

Renal column

Renal hilum

Renal pyramid

3rd lumbar vertebra

Renal medulla

Ureter

Renal papillae

Uterine tube

Area cribosa

Fimbria

Base of pyramid

Ovary

Descending colon

Uterus

Cervix

Endometrium

Sacrum

Myometrium

Sigmoid colon

Cervical canal

Urinary bladder

Vagina

Urine

Coccyx

Pubic bone

Rectum

Clitoris

Anus

Labium minus

Tendon levator ani

Labium majus

Vaginal opening

Urethra

Pelvic bone m.m.

LATERAL VIEW

RIGHT KIDNEY

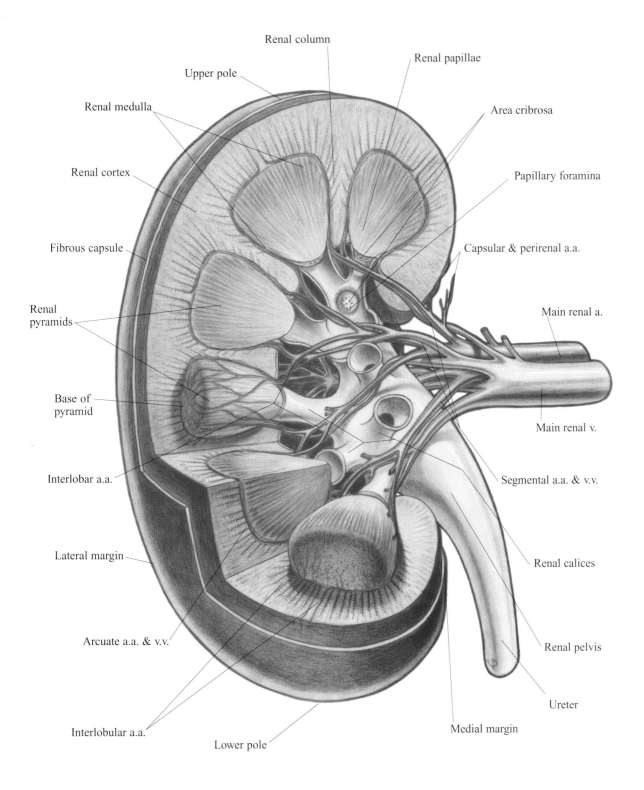

Renal column

Renal papillae

Upper pole

Renal medulla

Area cribrosa

Renal cortex

Papillary foramina

Fibrous capsule

Capsular & perirenal a.a.

Renal pyramids

Main renal a.

Base of pyramid

Main renal v.

Interlobar a.a.

Segmental a.a. & v.v.

Lateral margin

Renal calices

Arcuate a.a. & v.v.

Renal pelvis

Interlobular a.a.

Ureter

Lower pole

Medial margin

UROGENITAL SYSTEM

RENAL CORPUSCLE

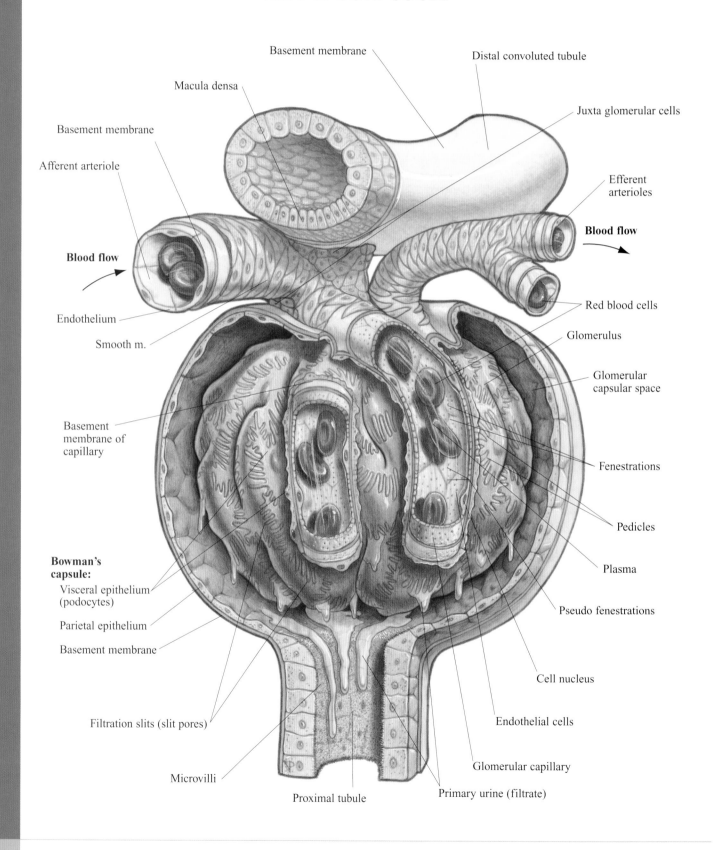

Basement membrane

Macula densa

Basement membrane

Afferent arteriole

Blood flow

Endothelium

Smooth m.

Basement
membrane of
capillary

**Bowman's
capsule:**

Visceral epithelium
(podocytes)

Parietal epithelium

Basement membrane

Filtration slits (slit pores)

Microvilli

Proximal tubule

Distal convoluted tubule

Juxta glomerular cells

Efferent
arterioles

Blood flow

Red blood cells

Glomerulus

Glomerular
capsular space

Fenestrations

Pedicles

Plasma

Pseudo fenestrations

Cell nucleus

Endothelial cells

Glomerular capillary

Primary urine (filtrate)

NEPHRON

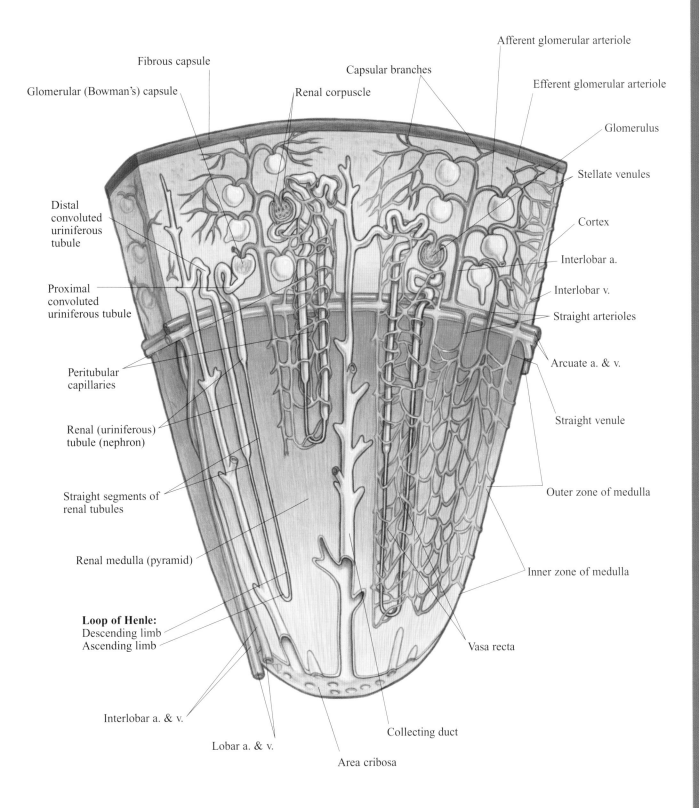

Fibrous capsule

Glomerular (Bowman's) capsule

Capsular branches

Renal corpuscle

Afferent glomerular arteriole

Efferent glomerular arteriole

Glomerulus

Stellate venules

Distal convoluted uriniferous tubule

Cortex

Interlobar a.

Proximal convoluted uriniferous tubule

Interlobar v.

Straight arterioles

Peritubular capillaries

Arcuate a. & v.

Renal (uriniferous) tubule (nephron)

Straight venule

Straight segments of renal tubules

Outer zone of medulla

Renal medulla (pyramid)

Inner zone of medulla

Loop of Henle:
Descending limb
Ascending limb

Vasa recta

Interlobar a. & v.

Lobar a. & v.

Collecting duct

Area cribosa

199

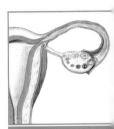

15

REPRODUCTIVE SYSTEM

MALE REPRODUCTIVE SYSTEM

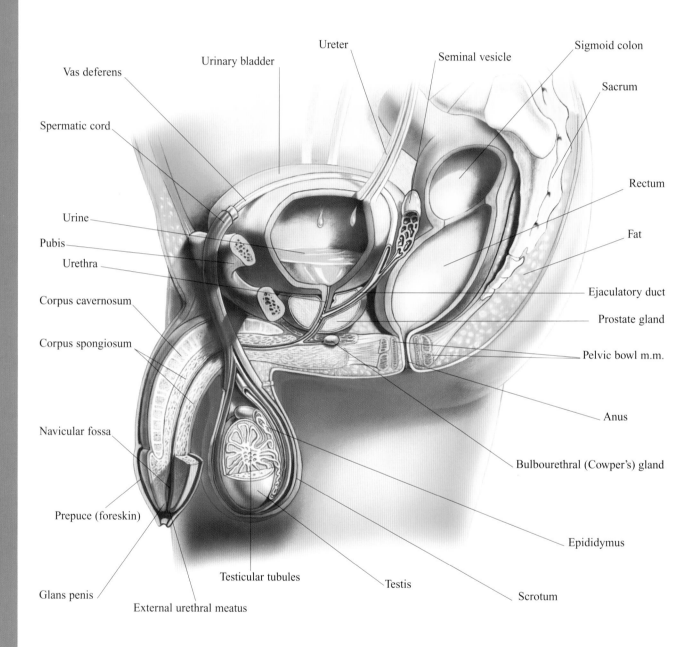

Vas deferens

Spermatic cord

Urine

Pubis

Urethra

Corpus cavernosum

Corpus spongiosum

Navicular fossa

Prepuce (foreskin)

Glans penis

External urethral meatus

Testicular tubules

Urinary bladder

Ureter

Seminal vesicle

Sigmoid colon

Sacrum

Rectum

Fat

Ejaculatory duct

Prostate gland

Pelvic bowl m.m.

Anus

Bulbourethral (Cowper's) gland

Epididymus

Testis

Scrotum

a.	=	**artery**
a.a.	=	**arteries**
L.	=	**Left**
l.	=	**ligament**
m.m.	=	**muscles**
R.	=	**Right**
v.	=	**vein**
v.v.	=	**veins**

FEMALE REPRODUCTIVE SYSTEM

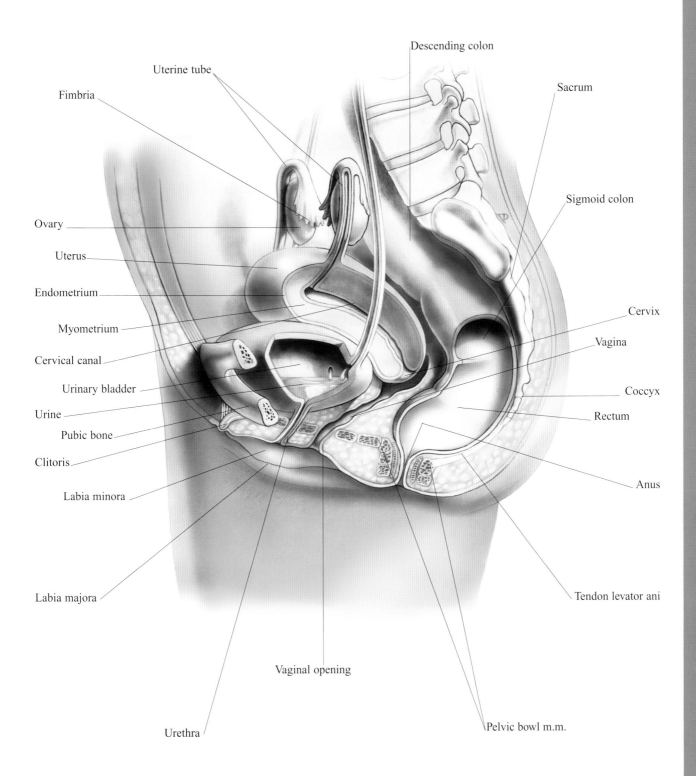

Descending colon

Uterine tube

Fimbria

Sacrum

Sigmoid colon

Ovary

Uterus

Endometrium

Cervix

Myometrium

Vagina

Cervical canal

Urinary bladder

Coccyx

Urine

Rectum

Pubic bone

Clitoris

Labia minora

Anus

Labia majora

Tendon levator ani

Vaginal opening

Urethra

Pelvic bowl m.m.

STAGES OF SPERM & OVUM

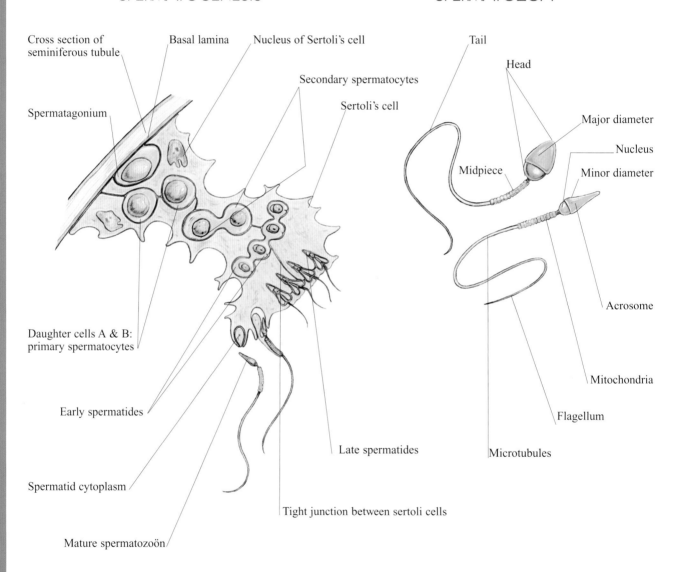

SPERMATOGENESIS

Cross section of
seminiferous tubule

Basal lamina

Nucleus of Sertoli's cell

Secondary spermatocytes

Spermatagonium

Sertoli's cell

Daughter cells A & B:
primary spermatocytes

Early spermatides

Spermatid cytoplasm

Late spermatides

Tight junction between sertoli cells

Mature spermatozoön

SPERMATOZOA

Tail

Head

Major diameter

Nucleus

Minor diameter

Midpiece

Acrosome

Mitochondria

Flagellum

Microtubules

STAGES OF SPERM & OVUM

OVUM

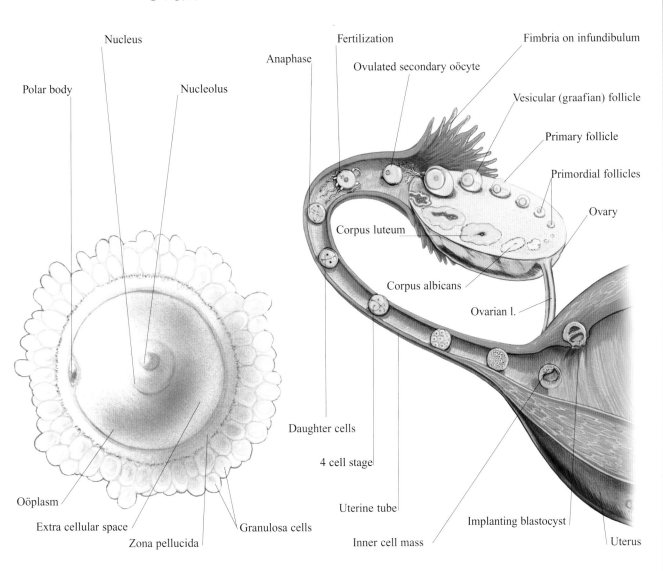

Nucleus

Polar body

Nucleolus

Anaphase

Fertilization

Ovulated secondary oöcyte

Fimbria on infundibulum

Vesicular (graafian) follicle

Primary follicle

Primordial follicles

Ovary

Corpus luteum

Corpus albicans

Ovarian l.

Daughter cells

4 cell stage

Uterine tube

Implanting blastocyst

Inner cell mass

Uterus

Oöplasm

Extra cellular space

Zona pellucida

Granulosa cells

UTERINE CYCLE

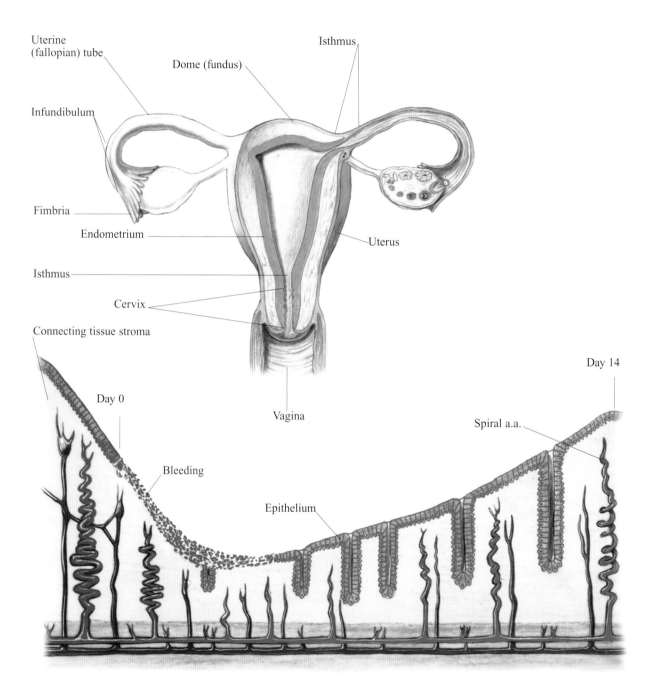

Uterine (fallopian) tube

Dome (fundus)

Isthmus

Infundibulum

Fimbria

Endometrium

Uterus

Isthmus

Cervix

Connecting tissue stroma

Day 14

Day 0

Spiral a.a.

Bleeding

Epithelium

Vagina

UTERINE CYCLE

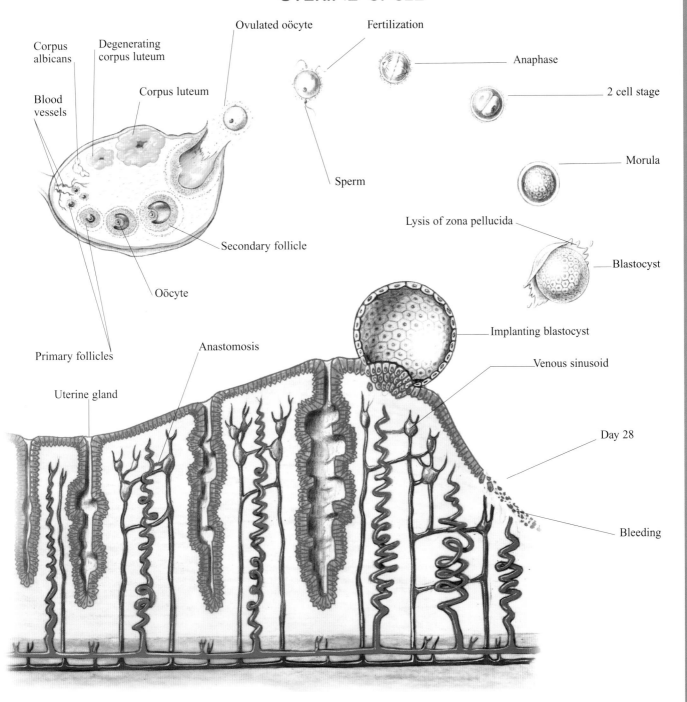

Ovulated oöcyte

Fertilization

Anaphase

2 cell stage

Corpus albicans

Degenerating corpus luteum

Corpus luteum

Blood vessels

Morula

Sperm

Lysis of zona pellucida

Secondary follicle

Blastocyst

Oöcyte

Implanting blastocyst

Primary follicles

Anastomosis

Venous sinusoid

Uterine gland

Day 28

Bleeding

FETAL CIRCULATION

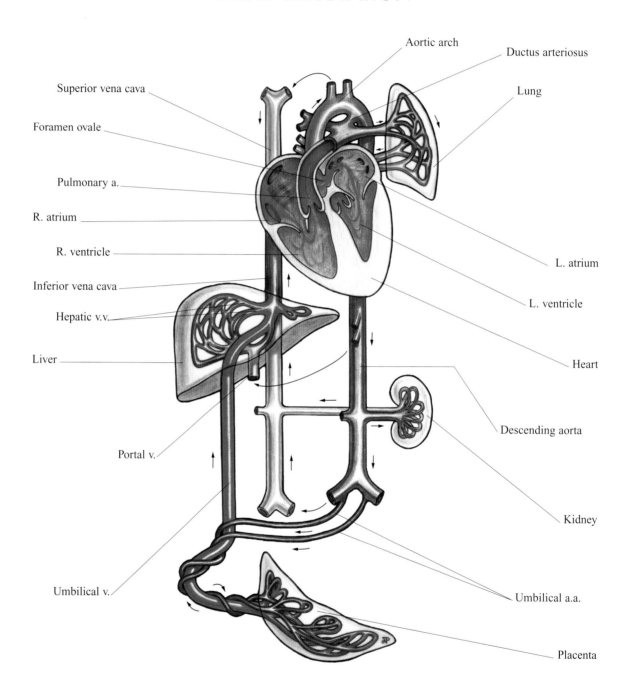

Aortic arch

Ductus arteriosus

Superior vena cava

Lung

Foramen ovale

Pulmonary a.

R. atrium

R. ventricle

L. atrium

Inferior vena cava

L. ventricle

Hepatic v.v.

Heart

Liver

Descending aorta

Portal v.

Kidney

Umbilical v.

Umbilical a.a.

Placenta

red	= oxygenated blood
blue	= unoxygenated blood
violet	= mixed blood

FULL-TERM BABY

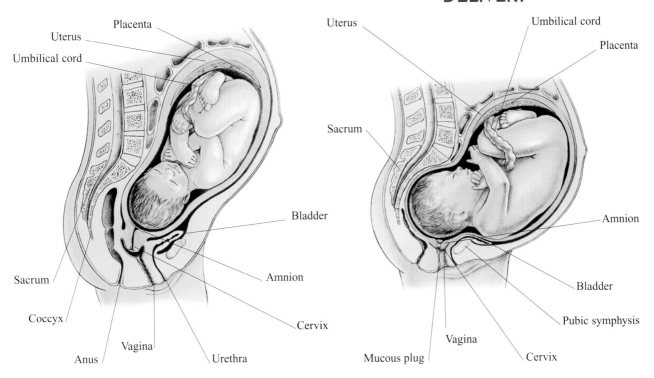

Uterus
Placenta
Umbilical cord

Bladder

Sacrum

Coccyx

Anus

Vagina

Urethra

Amnion

Cervix

FULL-TERM BABY PRIOR TO DELIVERY

Uterus
Umbilical cord
Placenta

Sacrum

Amnion

Bladder

Pubic symphysis

Mucous plug

Vagina

Cervix

FULL-TERM BABY BEING DELIVERED

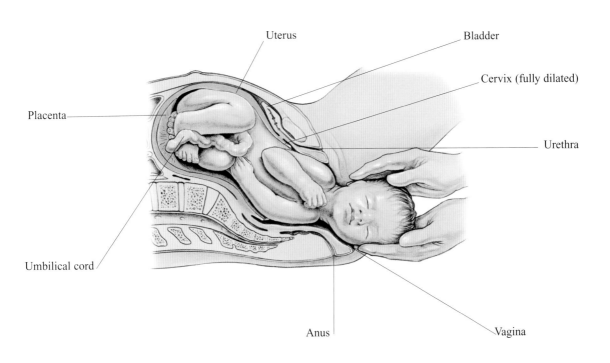

Uterus
Bladder

Cervix (fully dilated)

Placenta

Urethra

Umbilical cord

Anus

Vagina

SEXUAL INTERCOURSE

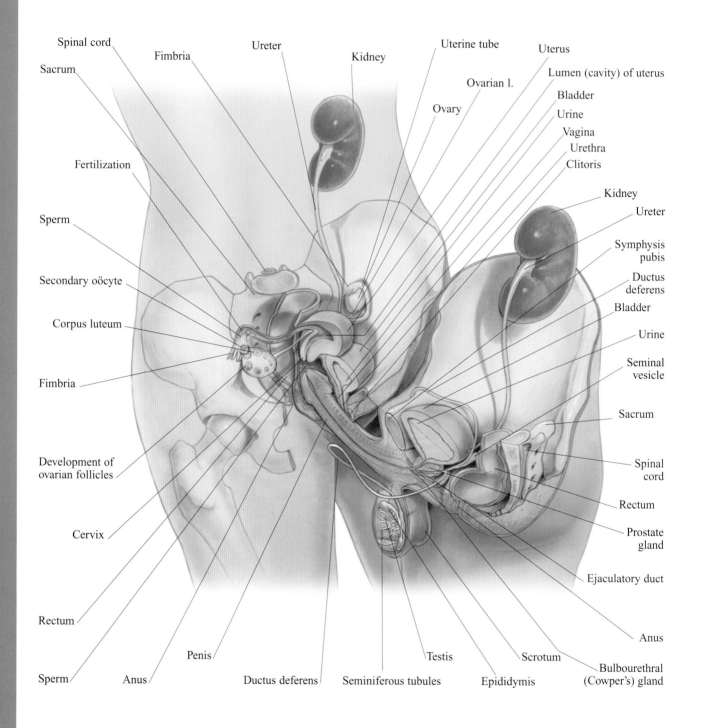

Spinal cord

Sacrum

Fimbria

Ureter

Kidney

Uterine tube

Uterus

Fertilization

Sperm

Secondary oöcyte

Corpus luteum

Fimbria

Development of
ovarian follicles

Cervix

Rectum

Sperm

Anus

Penis

Ductus deferens

Seminiferous tubules

Testis

Epididymis

Scrotum

Bulbourethral
(Cowper's) gland

Ovarian l.

Ovary

Lumen (cavity) of uterus

Bladder

Urine

Vagina

Urethra

Clitoris

Kidney

Ureter

Symphysis
pubis

Ductus
deferens

Bladder

Urine

Seminal
vesicle

Sacrum

Spinal
cord

Rectum

Prostate
gland

Ejaculatory duct

Anus

NOTES

INDEX

INDEX

INDEX

INDEX